Telling Is
Risky Business

Telling Is Risky Business

Mental Health Consumers Confront Stigma

Otto F. Wahl

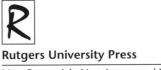

Rutgers University Press

New Brunswick, New Jersey, and London

148344

Library of Congress Cataloging-in-Publication Data

Wahl, Otto F.
    Telling is risky business : mental health consumers confront
stigma / Otto F. Wahl.
        p. cm.
    Includes bibliographical references and index.
    ISBN 0-8135-2723-6 (cl. : alk. paper). — ISBN 0-8135-2724-4 (pbk. :
alk. paper)
       1. Mental illness—Public opinion. 2. Psychiatry—Public opinion.
3. Stigma (Social psychology) I. Title.
RC454.4.W327 2000
362.2—dc21   99-18360
                                                  CIP

British Cataloging-in-Publication data for this book is available from the British
Library.

Manufactured in the United States of America

With thanks to my wife, Anne,
who found me the space to write,
and to my special Goops, whose
chair saved my knees while I wrote

Contents

Foreword

At the close of the twentieth century and what has been deemed "The Decade of the Brain," people with certain brain disorders—schizophrenia, bipolar disorder, major depression, and others—are arguably the last group of individuals who, by virtue of an illness, are socially outcast. It is still socially acceptable for cartoonists, policy-makers, health-care professionals, and the public-at-large to mock, stereotype, avoid, and otherwise denigrate people who experience a mental illness.

To be sure, palpable progress has been made against the stigmatization and discrimination of people with mental illnesses. Witness an October 1998 episode of the prime-time television series *Chicago Hope*, which portrayed a man with a severe mental illness as sympathetic and deserving of optimal treatment: on this program a doctor fought an HMO representative for access to a new antipsychotic medication, even though it was more expensive than the older and less effective medication on the company's formulary. Look at some leading opinion-page writers, such as Frank Rich with the *New York Times* and the nationally syndicated Richard Estado, who now routinely speak out on behalf of those who experience these brain diseases. Many writers have come forth with personal stories of mental illness, such as the powerful Katharine Graham, publisher of the *Washington Post*, in her 1997 award-winning and best-selling autobiography, *Personal History*. In September 1998, the *Oprah Winfrey Show* featured Wally Lamb and his *I Know This Much Is True*, a book describing a family confronting schizophrenia. The book is achingly realistic, and the segment of *Oprah* raised a strongly sympathetic voice, with video clips of consumers themselves. You know times are a-changing when, on the floor of the U.S. Senate, four U.S. senators—Domenici, Wellstone, Conrad, and Simpson—speaking in April 1996 on behalf of health insurance parity, recounted dramatically and publicly their personal brushes with mental illness. Even media coverage of high-profile murder cases involving individuals with severe mental illnesses—such as Russell Westin, accused of the July 1998 killing of two U.S. Capitol Police guards, and Michael Lauder, accused of killing his fiancee in New York in June 1998—showed greater recognition of the medical nature of the illness involved and the impact of the illness on the individuals and their families; this depiction led at least one journalist on the *Larry King Live* show to characterize coverage of the Lauder incident as a turning point in media coverage of mental illness and violent crime.

But with these gains persist the harsh and heartbreaking reality of pervasive scorn for individuals with psychiatric disorders. In the September 1998 issue of the *Journal of Occupational and Environmental Medicine*, researchers reported that employers are much less likely to hire someone who recently suffered a bout of depression versus equally qualified individuals with another medical illness. Almost 60 percent of the eighty personnel directors interviewed said they would never choose a candidate with depression for an executive job, versus 3 percent who said they would never hire a person with diabetes for such a position. Protests by residents of an affluent Washington, D.C., suburb against the opening of a group home for people with mental disabilities in their neighborhood were a topic of a National Public Radio discussion during 1998. Dr. Kay Jamison, the prolific mental illness researcher and author who courageously revealed her own struggle with bipolar disorder, has publicly disclosed the animus directed toward her by some members of her own profession—that is, mental health professionals—as a result of her revelation.

So even as we witness important high water marks in the way mental illness is discussed, the message has not filtered down to the everyday person in the workplace, on the street where you live, and the health-care professional. Truth be told, the media's coverage of mental illness and policies affecting people with these illnesses are still largely stigmatizing and discriminatory, respectively. Most people are still covered by health insurance that lacks equal coverage of mental illness treatment with other medical care. Research data, in fact, show that, since passage of a landmark federal bill in 1996 outlawing certain forms of insurance limits on mental illness treatment, insurance companies and HMOs have applied other measures to limit access to mental illness treatment.

The research eloquently described in this book documents the ongoing problems of stigma, and, unlike so many of its predecessors, it goes right to the horse's mouth—individuals who themselves have a serious mental illness. Dr. Wahl respectfully records the impressions, experiences, and views of those who are so scandalously treated by our society. And their testimony is the best bellwether of mental illness stigma. They tell us about the loneliness of mental illnesses, the social rejection, the ridicule undermining of their aspirations and work toward recovery, and the familiar name-calling and patronization. They testify to a constant war against them as human beings, a war in which they are too often beaten down and surrender their very beliefs in themselves. They recount the injustice of their treatment, and the ensuing suffering—not only because of an illness but also because of our lack of knowledge and compassion and our inherent meanness as a society.

Maybe you don't believe that things are really that bad. But our views of mental illness and the action they permit or produce are literally killing people with these diseases.

A 1998 investigative series, conducted by *The Hartford Courant*, found that, during the past decade, literally hundreds of people with mental illnesses were killed or severely harmed in hospitals, where they were brutally secluded or restrained; this treatment reflects the poor staffing, training, and funding made available for mental health treatment and our communal tolerance of mistreatment. We do not even require that statistics on such deaths be kept on a regular basis. One vignette from the *Courant* series typifies the horror (K. Mega and D. F. Blint, "Little Training, Few Standards, Poor Staffing Put Lives at Risk," October 12, 1998):

> She was a 15–year-old patient, alone in a new and frightening
>   place, clutching a comforting picture from home.
> He was a 200–pound mental health aide bent on enforcing

the rules, and the rules said no pictures. She defied him;
the dispute escalated.
And for that, Edith Campos died. She was crushed face down
on the floor in a "therapeutic hold" applied by a man twice
her size.

We should be ashamed, as a society, of treating individuals in
such a way. Our shame should be compounded by the fact that this
mistreatment is unnecessary and wasteful. We are living in an age
when treatments for mental illnesses are better than ever before. Most
consumers today actually enjoy the prospect of much diminished
disability and even full recovery. By virtue of biomedical advances
and innovations in community treatment approaches, most people
with mental disorders can look forward to a real life—a meaningful,
productive, self-directed life.

In a strange way, prevailing stigmas against people with mental
illnesses prevent us from dealing with the very problems we so fear.
Although most individuals with serious mental illnesses are no more
violent than the general population, for a small minority without
treatment and often with a co-occurring substance-abuse problem,
violent actions do occur. In addition, some of the most ill individuals, in episodes of intense symptoms, can indeed look unkempt.
Unfortunately, as society broadly applies this image to everyone with
a mental illness, advocates for those with psychiatric disorders too
often find it too damaging to take up such difficult issues and work
toward solution. The solution is, generally, access to treatment—
something a society that discriminates against people with mental
illnesses is too stingy to assure.

It is time that our viewpoints and policies become aligned with
the medical progress we have thankfully witnessed. In this book the
voices of the brave consumers—individuals who have suffered so
much but have refused to be denied a life with dignity and purpose—
enjoin us to end discrimination against mental illness once and for
all.

I am very heartened by the work that is presented in this book. It
tells an incredibly important story about what is and what can be for
people with mental illnesses. This book will likely open your eyes to

a topic you probably did not understand. It will lead you to admire individuals who have struggled against great odds. It presents the voices of people who have mounted the struggle and hopefully will lead you to the belief that we cannot as a people tolerate further cruelty and discrimination against these, our sons and daughters, brothers and sisters, mothers and fathers, neighbors, and fellow citizens.

Laura Lee Hall, Ph.D.
Director of Research
NAMI (formerly National Alliance for the Mentally Ill)

Preface

Ted Kaczynski, the alleged Unabomber, made very clear that he would rather risk the death penalty than employ a more promising defense that argued he had a mental illness.[1] He appeared not to mind being known as a killer, but he strongly resisted being labeled mentally ill.

Although Martha Stewart no doubt handles most criticism with the graciousness of a good hostess, when the *National Enquirer* suggested that she was mentally ill, the air quickly became filled with talk of lawsuits.[2] People agreed that her reputation was greatly besmirched by such a suggestion and that Ms. Stewart could easily have been emotionally damaged by such a harsh and undeserved indictment.

"When my depression was first diagnosed," wrote Kathy Cronkite, "I felt both relief and shame—relief that my condition was real, had a name, and possibly a cure; shame that I was afflicted with a mental disorder. I still felt I should have been able to rise above it, to use my will to overcome it on my own, and that my inability to do so was proof of my weak nature. I kept the diagnosis and my condition a secret from all but my husband and family, at first."[3]

When history scholars proposed that the body of famous explorer Meriwether Lewis be exhumed to verify reports that he had taken his own life, there was substantial resistance. This resistance was not based solely on moral or emotional reactions to disturbing the body; instead, some people feared the possible harm to Lewis's reputation should it be conclusively established that depression led him to commit suicide. A reporter in the *Washington Post* argued, for example, that Lewis could not have been mentally ill because "by temperament, he was a fighter, not a quitter," as if succumbing to depression represented a lack of resolve or will or character. A forensic scientist in that same article is quoted as lamenting that "the taint of suicide is very distinct on [Lewis's] reputation."[4]

Robert Boorstin—presidential aide, special assistant to the secretary of state, and a sufferer from manic-depressive disorder—has observed: "I used to think a lot when I was a kid about running for office, when I was a teenager and when I was in college. After I got sick, all those thoughts went away. If I was to stand for office, even a local office somewhere, I could be labeled as nuts, crazy. The stigma could completely wipe out any chance that I had of doing something for a community."[5]

All of these circumstances are manifestations of the stigma of mental illness, the burdensome phenomenon with which this book is concerned. In fact, some mental health consumers, such as Barbara Brundage, have described stigma as "the hardest thing for me to overcome," worse even than mental illness itself.[6] The National Institute of Mental Health, likewise, has noted that the stigma of mental illness "becomes [consumers'] most debilitating handicap."[7] Mental illness stigma, moreover, is a phenomenon that is likely to affect us all.

This latter assertion is based on the fact that mental illness is *not* a rare phenomenon that happens to only a few vulnerable individuals. Epidemiological studies have established that about one in every one hundred American adults will suffer from schizophrenia, one in every one hundred will have bipolar (manic-depressive) disorder, one in every one hundred will struggle with profound depression, and one in every two hundred persons will contend with obsessive-compulsive disorder. Overall, estimates from available studies are that from 20 to almost 50 percent of the adult population of the United States will suffer a diagnosable psychiatric disorder at some time in their lives.[8] This large number will include doctors and lawyers, teachers and students, pilots and pianists, millionaires and paupers, conferring immunity on no one by virtue of their financial, educational, or cultural advantage. In addition, even more individuals will be affected by psychiatric disorders through their contact with friends, relatives, neighbors, and coworkers who have mental illnesses. Many times those with mental illness will be people about whom we care deeply—our children, parents, spouses, lifelong friends.

The need both to understand mental disorders and to facilitate the recovery of those who are afflicted with them is important to us all.

It is unfortunate, however, that mental illness is not only common but also misunderstood. In a 1990 telephone survey conducted by the Daniel Yanklovich Group on behalf of the Robert Wood Johnson Foundation, a representative sample of the U.S. population reported that they felt better informed about all other health problems tested (alcoholism, cancer, drug abuse, heart disease, and AIDS) than they did about mental illness. Only 25 percent were able to describe themselves as "very well informed" about mental illness, and 60 percent agreed that they should know more about it.[9] In the absence of adequate knowledge about mental illness, misconceptions abound. A 1996 survey of slightly more than one thousand Americans, for example, revealed that 31 to 41 percent of respondents believed that chronic depression and schizophrenia are due to weakness in personal character.[10] Such misconceptions contribute to highly unfavorable views of the people who experience such disorders; these views, in turn, create a countertherapeutic environment that undermines efforts to cope with and recover from mental illness. *Stigma* is the term that represents these negative and inaccurate views of mental illness, and, just as mental illness affects millions of us and our friends and loved ones, so too does the mental illness stigma. Motivation for understanding and caring about the stigma experienced by mental health consumers, then, can come from more than just human empathy for suffering strangers (though such empathy is surely to be desired); it is demanded by the reality that such stigma harms those we know and care about, if not ourselves.

As readers may have already observed, individuals who have had mental illness, psychiatric treatment, or diagnoses of mental disorder are referred to in this book as "consumers," and some discussion of the choice of that term is in order. There is continuing debate over what to call those who have experienced psychiatric disorders, and, as we do with other distinct groups in society, I have tried to be guided by what those groups prefer to be called. With respect to mental illness, there is not complete consensus. Indeed, a 1996 study of 302 participants in psychiatric treatment programs found no one term to be preferred by the majority of the study respondents.[11] Many people with psychiatric disorders, however, are quite clear that they find their previous designations as "patients" unacceptable; they see the term as implying that they are diseased and passive recipients of the ministrations of powerful doctors assigned to fix them. Some object to the terms "mental illness" or "psychiatric disorder" as applied to them for similar reasons. Some have expressed preference for terms like "psychiatric survivor" to indicate that they have managed to go on despite their devastating illnesses—or even to suggest that they have survived the terrors and indignities of psychiatric treatment.

One of the most widely used and widely accepted terms within the community of advocates with previous psychiatric treatment is "consumer of mental health services" or "mental health consumer."[12] Although some still object to the term—for example, as suggesting that they are merely takers who consume resources and give nothing back—the term "consumer" is intended to convey that the individual with mental illness is an active participant in the treatment process, selecting and negotiating for the best services and/or products, as do respected consumers of other products in our society. Many of the leading organizations of people with mental illnesses have chosen the term "consumer" for themselves—such as the National Mental Health Consumers Self-Help Clearinghouse and the Consumer Council of NAMI (formerly known as the National Alliance for the Mentally Ill).[13] Accordingly, in the study described in this book, and throughout the book, the term "consumer" is used as a convenient and reasonably well-accepted shorthand for a person identified or diagnosed as having a psychiatric disorder.

Whatever nomenclature one chooses, consumers, patients, survivors constitute the focus of this book. Understanding stigma—how it is manifest, what obstacles it poses for those with mental illnesses, and what is its impact on the individual—is an important first step toward overcoming it. One key to that understanding is to hear from consumers who may have experienced stigma, to find out what they have experienced and how they have reacted to it: Those with psychiatric disorders can best enlighten us about the reactions they have received. The sufferers of mental illness can best convey what their illnesses have meant to them. The consumers working toward recovery can best tell us what barriers stigma has created for them.

The purpose of the current book, then, is to examine and summarize what mental health consumers have to say about their experiences of stigma so that public and professional understanding may be increased. At the center of this examination are the results of a yearlong, nationwide study in which consumers were asked to tell about their experiences of stigma and discrimination, through both questionnaires and interviews. I have done my best in this book to pass on what consumers told us in this study, along with what has been communicated and learned from other similar opportunities for consumers to report their experiences. As noted in chapter 3, consumers were eager to talk with us and finally tell their stories. What they told us was both enlightening and, at times, discouraging. As someone who has long studied and discussed mental illness stigma, I was not entirely surprised by the responses I received; however, even I could not help but be moved, angered, educated, and occasionally embarrassed by what I was told. Consumers, moreover, told their stories with passion and insight, and I did not want to merely digest their words into stale summaries. Therefore, to afford readers as realistic an appreciation of consumers' experiences as possible, I have included many quotations from consumers. I hope that those direct statements may help the readers of this book to appreciate consumers' experiences of stigma in the same way that their stories have helped me to better appreciate what they face every day.

Mental illness and mental illness stigma occur in the context of a whole life. They occur to unique individuals with families and personalities and aspirations, a fact sometimes lost in a sole focus on experiences that occur after the onset of mental illness. Thus, chapter 1 presents a detailed account of one particular individual whose story, it is hoped, reminds readers of the persons behind the accounts of stigma to be presented in subsequent chapters. Chapter 2 then reviews the general concept of stigma and prior research investigating public attitudes and reactions toward mental illness. This research has demonstrated the fertile ground for stigma experiences (widespread negative public attitudes and misconceptions) but, for the most part, has neglected to talk to consumers about what they have actually encountered.[14] In chapter 3, I describe the central study's development and implementation in order to allow as many consumers as possible to provide input about their experiences. The characteristics of those consumers responding are detailed, and the chapter also includes participants' comments that demonstrate their eagerness to be heard and included. The following chapters summarize the main experiences reported by study respondents: being isolated and rejected by others (chapter 4), facing discouragement about their potential for accomplishment from others (chapter 5), being discriminated against and denied opportunities on the basis of their psychiatric history (chapter 6), witnessing mental illness being discussed and depicted by others in offensive and demeaning ways (chapter 7), and worrying about what may happen if their treatment histories are disclosed or discovered (chapter 8). The harmful effects that these experiences have had on consumers—on self-esteem, motivation, opportunity, and recovery—are considered in chapter 8 as well.

Consumers interviewed as part of the study were asked to describe both their strategies to cope with stigma and their suggestions to reduce such stigma; their ideas are described in chapter 9. Interviewees were also given the opportunity to articulate messages they would like to give to the public about mental illness; chapter 10 describes those messages. Like all research studies, ours has a number of limitations; those limitations and some cautions about interpretation of results are conveyed in chapter 11. Chapter 12 provides a list of resources for those interested in further information about mental illnesses and, in particular, about the personal experiences of those who have had psychiatric disorders. Finally, several appendices provide copies of the survey questionnaire, characteristics of survey participants, and tabular summaries of responses.

I am indebted to many people for their assistance in completing this project. First, NAMI provided generous funding for the study of consumer experiences of stigma as part of their important Campaign to End Discrimination Against People with Brain Disorders. NAMI staff also contributed time, assistance, and valuable advice in carrying out the study. I am grateful to Mike Malloy, Ferrell Fitch, and Maggie Scheie-Lurie for both their enthusiasm and their continuing help on the research, and especially to Laura Lee Hall for both her help in completing the study and her willingness to write the foreword to this book. In addition, Frieda Eastman was instrumental in getting our survey questionnaire published in the NAMI newsletter, *The Advocate*, as was Barbara Hoopes in posting the survey on NAMI's internet site. Volunteers from NAMI's Consumer Council were helpful in the feedback they provided on early drafts of the study questionnaire and in distributing the survey in their home locales.

Numerous students from George Mason University were of assistance as well. Clinical psychology doctoral students Dina Wiecynski, Mark Gruber, Jenny Tsai, and Candi Reinsmith worked many hours coding and recording survey responses, conducting, transcribing, and coding interviews, and assisting in data analysis. The daunting task of transcribing one hundred hours of interviews was undertaken also by additional graduate and undergraduate volunteers, including Barbara Evans, Bertille Donohoe, Jessica Morvan, Bridget Peach, Jennifer Gay, and Na-Youg Yoo. In addition, we were fortunate to have Susan Lewis, herself a mental health consumer, volunteer her expertise in computer science to help us manage the large amount of data we accumulated and to help us tame the computer systems that sometimes seemed decidedly uncooperative.

Finally, I must thank the approximately fourteen hundred mental health consumers who took the time to respond to our survey and to the one hundred who talked with us at length over the telephone about their experiences. I am particularly grateful to Dorene Sherman; she not only agreed to have the details of her life described in chapter 1 so that others might better understand what life is like for a person with mental illness, but she also courageously declined anonymity to be sure that she did not perpetuate stigma by behaving as if her illness were something one should be ashamed to admit. Consumers like Dorene, and the many others who provided us with information, are, in fact, the most important figures in this book, for their experiences—sometimes sad, sometimes infuriating, and mostly courageous—serve as the core of this book and lead us to a fuller understanding of mental illness stigma and what it does.

Telling Is
Risky Business

1

One Person's

Story

Dorene Sherman is a thirty-five-year-old woman who has lived most of her life in and around Toledo, Ohio. Raised primarily by her mother and grandmother, she maintains close ties with both. Dorene is also a single parent of a seven-year-old boy with whom she especially enjoys reading and playing baseball. She likes bluegrass music and plays both the clarinet and the mandolin. She has organized conferences, given speeches before large groups, and contributed extensively as a Democratic campaign worker. In May 1998, she completed her master's degree in counseling at Heidelberg College and then gained employment as an extended care worker in the Christian school her son was attending. Dorene Sherman has also struggled with mental illness for most of her life.

Dorene's parents were divorced when she was around three years of age. Nevertheless, Dorene recalls her early family life as being relatively happy. She remembers going to drive-in movies with her mother and spending much pleasant time at her grandmother's house in Toledo while her mom worked. In fact, her memories of her time at her grandmother's are extremely positive. "That house," she says, "was where I wanted to be. . . . Everything was at that house and that's the best part of any of my childhood memories that I have." Dorene is pleased to report that she and her mother and grandmother continue to share a home.

Dorene recalls two female friends who lived on her street and played with her often. However, she also recollects feeling somewhat isolated as a child and finding it difficult to get close to those outside her family. "I used to look at it that I was doing something that was going to screw everything up. . . . I worried about them getting angry with me and never coming back." As a result, she often "backed off" from other people.

Dorene has mixed recollections of her grade school experiences as well. As a good student she brought home good grades, even in what later became her major stumbling block—math. And she had a third-grade teacher whom she really liked and who liked her as well. Although she did not like to think of herself as "teacher's pet," that is, she says, what she became. "I felt really comfortable with her, and she liked me too. . . . She used to give me privileges to take something down to the principal. And I don't remember doing anything special. It was kind of like I connected onto her and really liked her. And it was kind of the same [for her] with me." This teacher, only a substitute, moved on to a different job and left Dorene so emotionally saddened by her departure that other children began to make fun of her by saying she was "acting like she was my mother or something."

Life really began to unravel for Dorene starting in junior high school. Although she had started out as a thin child, Dorene began to put on weight. She recalls, in fact, that, by age nine, she was on a Weight Watchers program. In seventh grade, Dorene and her mother moved to a new school system outside of Toledo where, as a new and somewhat overweight student, she was teased by her schoolmates about her appearance. "I wasn't terribly obese in seventh grade," she remembers, "but I was, you know, bigger, a big kid. And kids used to make fun of me. I remember crying and wanting to go back to school in Toledo and go back and live in my grandma's house." In this atmosphere, her grades began to go down. Instead of As and Bs, Dorene got Cs and Ds. Math proved especially difficult and remained so for her through high school and beyond.

Concerns about her weight and appearance escalated to a point where, by sophomore year in high school, Dorene had a full-fledged eating disorder, where she binged and purged more and more frequently. At the same time, she began experiencing mood swings. "My moods would change all over the place," she recalls. "First I would eat. I would eat and eat and eat. And then I would sleep. I would want to sleep. . . . I wanted to be in the bed and I couldn't get out of the bed." Dorene began to miss school and, on occasion, even purposely cut herself so badly that she required stitches (although she always told people it had been an accident).

Dorene also describes, with some embarrassment, her creation of an imaginary friend as part of her struggle for acceptance: "When I was in high school, I would pretend that I had a friend, and the friend didn't really exist at all, and I would tell my friends about this person, and my friends would want to meet this person and I would really build this friend up, 'cause this friend was really cool and this friend really liked me. And it got to a point where the kids, the kids knew."

In the midst of all of this, however, Dorene nevertheless found some sources of satisfaction. She took up the clarinet and found that she was quickly able to learn to play. (Later she became interested in bluegrass music when her mother married a man who had grown up in Kentucky and Tennessee, and she took up the mandolin as well.) Dorene then became a member of the school band, which was "the one place I felt that I belonged. Because if you were a band person . . . everyone else thought you were weird, and we thought everyone else was weird. So I had my little place, finally." As a member of the marching band, Dorene joined others in playing at the school football games, performing in concerts, and participating in marching band competitions. Her musical talent extended to singing as well, and Dorene sang in the chorus for school functions. She has no hesitation in identifying her musical activities as a source of great satisfaction and pleasure for her. "I loved it," she recalls. "I loved it!"

Although her musical talents also permitted Dorene to earn better grades—As and Bs in band, for example—they did not spare her from further emotional struggles. She continued to binge and purge, and, at age nineteen, Dorene had her first psychiatric hospitalization, at which time she was diagnosed with bulimia. Despite the diagnosis and hospitalization, however, she became even more determined to control her weight through the use (and overuse) of laxatives. This led to repeated visits to emergency rooms and repeated hospitalizations, about three or four each year. As Dorene explained:

"I remember taking boxes of laxatives which actually was probably like seventy or eighty of them. And at that point I had already been binging and purging. So my potassium levels were really bad so that, when I would go in, I would end up being hooked up to an IV for a while. I always ended up on the psych floor. From the time that I was nineteen to when I was, probably, twenty-four or twenty-five, I was in and out all the time."

The treatment received while in the hospital was reportedly ineffective, in part because of Dorene's determination to keep her weight down. "I liked the way I looked at that point," she says, "and just liked being that way and I didn't care. . . . I figured I'm going to lose weight and I don't even care if it kills me." In part, though, Dorene did not improve because she found no programs specifically directed to her eating disorder. "The only treatment I got was get the potassium back in you, put you on the psych unit . . . until your insurance runs out, send you home for a while, then put you back in." Only later in her life, when she learned about an Eating Disorders Unit at a local hospital and entered that program, did Dorene begin to recover from her disorder. Even now, she says, the problem has never completely gone away.

The limitations of treatment imposed by health insurance coverage made a particular impression on Dorene. Her stays in the hospital, she recalls, would be about forty days, which was the length of stay covered by her insurance. In fact, she recalls being quite upset one time when she, having developed a good rapport with a particular doctor at the treatment clinic, was told that she would be unable to continue seeing him because her insurance had run out and she was being transferred to the state hospital.

Dorene does not remember clearly her reactions or her family's reactions to her psychiatric diagnosis and treatment. She recalls that when her stepfather told her the psychiatrist was going to keep her locked up until she stopped her binging and purging she began to lie to her family; she assured them that she was no longer binging even though the pattern continued. She does not recall being concerned about the reactions of her peers, although she did not want to see others when she was in the hospital: "At that time, I didn't mind if I was going to be up on a psych unit. I was just doing my thing, but I didn't want to see anybody. And, at that point, I still hadn't grasped that . . . people make fun of you."

Dorene also continued to have difficulty with mood swings. Most obvious were the "down" periods when she felt unable to get out of bed. But her more expansive moods led her to do things like spend lots of money, including that stolen from her mother's purse, and overcharging on credit cards. In her twenties, she also began drinking and partying, even though she had not been much of a drinker before. She recalls spending a good deal of time at a particular bar in Toledo where she would "binge drink." "I wouldn't drink every day, but, if I would go out, I wouldn't stop until I was like half dead." She and a friend would meet sailors, many from foreign countries, at the bar, eventually resulting in a bizarre incident in which Dorene brought home and married (and, shortly after, divorced) a sailor she had just met when he told her that he could not return to his ship or he would be beaten for being absent overnight. Other unusual behavior included her involvement with a drag queen and the gay subculture, as well as initial use of illegal drugs.

At the time, Dorene did not perceive these behaviors as a problem. "I wasn't in the hospital during this period. So I thought I was perfect. I thought I was doing wonderful 'cause I wasn't in the hospital." Other people viewed Dorene's behavior differently: some suggested that she was pretending when she claimed not to have energy; some just saw her as a "moody" or rebellious individual. As a result, Dorene received little additional help until she suffered a more significant and obvious breakdown.

As Dorene describes it, "I was getting into going a million miles an hour in the things I got involved in"—and there were many. In 1990, she became pregnant and gave birth to a son in May 1991. Later that year she returned to school and began volunteering to work on Bill Clinton's presidential campaign; she invested many hours in both school and campaign work in addition to her role as a single mother. Her apparent high energy earned her recognition as a dedicated campaign worker, and she was welcomed in the camp of other local politicians. "I had a real good reputation in the party," Dorene recounts. "I was one of the young Democrats that was coming up in the world. I had a bright future. I was going to do wonderful. I was Supermom.

And then, one day I was working on a campaign for someone running for Senate in Ohio . . . and I just totally lost it. I started crying and I was just hysterical." Taken to an emergency room, she was once again admitted to a psychiatric hospital where she was medicated and released in two weeks. Outside the hospital, she was depressed and again began to cut herself, which led to still another hospitalization. This time she was given a diagnosis of borderline personality disorder. No one, however, told her this diagnosis (she learned it, she recalls, only by seeing it on some paperwork being filed by the hospital). Nor was she told anything about the disorder from which she was supposedly suffering and for which, she reports, she received "a bazillion medications" that reduced her to a condition in which "I would just sleep and drool."

Fortunately, Dorene did have greater success with another therapist, one who charted her moods with her, identified her as suffering from bipolar (manic-depressive) disorder, and discussed with her that diagnosis and its treatment. With a more understanding and communicative therapist and with proper medications, Dorene has remained relatively stable for a number of years. However, she reports that "even when I'm stable, I'm still more active than the average person." In fact, she understands that she likes her high-energy states. "I like feeling active. I like it; people like it when I'm going a million miles an hour because I'm getting stuff done." She also admits that continuing to take her prescribed medication is sometimes difficult for her; it causes physical problems, such as diarrhea, and "makes me feel weird." Sometimes she neglects or forgets to take the medication. "And then my thoughts start getting messed up, and then I don't want to take it. I'm just like, well I'm doing fine and I don't need to take it." Her activity level increases, and she again goes "a million miles an hour" until she becomes exhausted and realizes she needs to spend a few days in a hospital with rest and medications to help her to become more stable once again. In recent years, however, she has rarely needed extended stays.

Dorene has, in fact, harnessed her energy to make substantial contributions in a variety of ways. She became involved with a group of other mental health consumers, the Consumers Union of Lucas County, Ohio, where she started out as a consumer advocate and soon became program coordinator. In these roles, she helped to establish support groups for consumers, assisted consumers in resolving landlord-tenant disputes, and visited hospitals to provide information on the work of the Consumers Union. Also instrumental in getting members of the Consumers Union to respond to the stigma survey discussed in this book, Dorene organized a conference on stigma at which I was able to report on the early results of the survey.

Dorene managed, furthermore, to complete both an undergraduate college degree and a master's degree in counseling. She hopes eventually to be employed in the mental health field. At the time she provided this information, however, she was working at her son's school as part of a very practical plan to enhance his education. To qualify for a discount on his tuition at the private Christian school—and to earn money beyond the Aid to Dependent Children and other support funds she receives—Dorene elected to work at the school as an extended care worker. With her typical high level of energy and achievement, she soon took over the position of extended care director.

Another primary area of Dorene's success—and a source of pride and pleasure—is her performance as a parent. "My son Jared," she says with obvious affection, "is the best thing that ever happened to me." Although she was in a manic phase when she became pregnant and actually remembers little about the circumstances of his birth, Dorene has no regrets about her decision to keep her son and raise him on her own. As a mother, she enjoys reading with him, playing in the park, and even just lounging around the house watching TV together. She tosses a baseball with him to indulge his interest in sports and takes him to movies when she can. Dorene worries, like most mothers, whether she is being a good parent, and her concerns are fueled by anxieties about how her psychiatric disorder might affect her son. "I used to think that he needed a better mother than me. Why should he have a mother who's sick and in the hospital?" Dorene even took Jared to her therapist to assess possible maladjustment resulting from her parenting. The therapist, as do most of Dorene's friends and colleagues, saw Jared as a bright, well-adjusted boy whose mother is doing a pretty good job raising a likeable young man.

Despite her many accomplishments, however, Dorene has been burdened by others' attitudes toward mental illness. As often happens to people with mental illness, she began to be treated differently when her illness became known to those with whom she worked. Although some of her coworkers showed much-appreciated understanding and sympathy, others did not. "When I got sick, a lot of these people who are leaders . . . got a little funny with me. They stayed, they were always very polite. The Young Dems, who I was the president [of] for a short time, they stopped talking to me." Like many other consumers who disclose their illnesses, she also found herself demoted to less demanding (and less satisfying) tasks: "It just made me feel bad, because I was once this bright and up-and-coming person, and now I'm the crazy person who sits over at the table over there licking the stamps."

Although she has generally found her church and people at her son's Christian school to be understanding and supportive, Dorene nevertheless was hurt by the reactions of a pastor when she was briefly hospitalized in 1998. At that time, the pastor visited her and, like many lay persons, seemed puzzled as to how a person as obviously intelligent and competent as she could need psychiatric care. He implied, according to Dorene, that "he wasn't sure if he believed in mental illness" and that "if I truly loved my job [working with children], then I wouldn't allow myself to get sick like that." Such remarks, although intended to be helpful, only made Dorene feel worse about needing treatment. "I'm telling myself, oh yeah, if I'm this and that and the other thing, then why am I sick?"

Dorene was also shocked and hurt by the attitudes and behavior she encountered in her counseling program when psychiatric disorders were discussed. She recalls people with mental illness being made fun of, for example. "This one woman who I've been through the whole entire program with, she was talking about a client that she had to do some personal care on" and presented this client in such a way that "the class was rolling over." She mentions numerous disparaging remarks about people with borderline personality disorder (one of her diagnoses); classmates made jokes about it and connected it laughingly to the Glenn Close character in the movie *Fatal Attraction*. Dorene also remembers confiding to her class instructor that she has bipolar disorder and being cautioned that, even in a class of people intending to work with those with psychiatric disorders, "you don't want to tell people that."

Insensitive media depiction of mental illness provided Dorene with one of her most memorable encounters with stigma. She was sitting in a movie theater with her then six-year old son watching *Good Burger*, a film based on the characters in a popular Nickelodeon children's show, *Keenan and Kel*. The comedy was silly enough to appeal to her young son, and she was enjoying their outing. About two-thirds of the way through the film, however, the action shifted to "Demented Hills Asylum" where patients in this fictional mental hospital included a man who ate the cards people were trying to use in a card game, another man who kept hitting his head with a ping-pong paddle, and a large, menacing man in a straitjacket who growled and glared rather than speak. All were dressed in drab, gray uniforms and surrounded by burly attendants/guards in white suits. Dorene was shocked and uncertain what to do. Her son knew that she had been in a psychiatric hospital, and she worried what he might be thinking. Did he think that this was the way she looked and acted, that this was the way she was treated? Would he connect what he was seeing with his mother's hospitalization and be upset or frightened or embarrassed? Should she leave the movie and perhaps deprive her child of an experience he appeared to be enjoying? Or should she stay and take the chance of his getting wrong and potentially upsetting ideas about her illness? She was also troubled by the fact that most of the theater audience was laughing about the mentally ill characters, and she did not want her son to accept the view that people with mental illnesses are to be ridiculed and laughed at.

To her credit, Dorene handled the situation probably as well as she could have. She first turned to her son and explained to him how it was not right to laugh at the people depicted on the screen: "I said, 'Do you remember when Mommy had to go to the hospital because the chemicals in her brain aren't working right? That's the same with those people, and everybody's making fun of them.' So then he connected with what was going on, and he stopped." After the movie, she initiated a long talk with her son, during which she explained how her experiences were different from those shown in the movie and how most people in mental hospitals were not like the ones in the film. No doubt her son benefited from both her openness and her controlled, educational response to the negative stereotypes of mental illness provided by the film.

Dorene's story is, in most ways, a consumer success story. Her disorder is under control, although it is not "cured," and Dorene still has to watch herself carefully to be sure that her activity does not become overactivity. Occasionally, as in the week before her interview for this book, she needs to return to the hospital to regain lost equilibrium. Nevertheless, Dorene has moved ahead with her life, continues to make substantial contributions to her family and her community, and has earned the respect of friends and coworkers for her dedication, efficiency, and parental caring. She cannot quite shake the stigma of mental illness, however, and continues to encounter, from time to time, hurtful and offensive attitudes and behavior that impede her recovery by both adding stress and undermining her already fragile self-esteem.

Those kinds of stigma experiences provided the basis for the study described in this book. Moreover, those kinds of experiences are recounted in subsequent chapters by hundreds of people who, like Dorene, struggle with illnesses they did not choose to have. As readers learn about the stigma and discrimination experiences that present the focus of this book, I hope that they will remember that the people to whom these experiences have occurred are far more than either the sum of those occurrences or their mental illness symptoms. They are, like Dorene Sherman, complex individuals who occupy multiple roles. They are parents and spouses and neighbors and coworkers. They are individuals with strengths as well as frailties, with abilities and aspirations, with human needs for affection, respect, admiration, and opportunity. They are people, like Dorene Sherman, who deserve our efforts to understand the experiences that they have taken the time and effort to communicate to us and that I attempt to pass on to the readers in the following chapters.

2

Mental Illness

Stigma

"Sylvia obviously was a person who was capable of feeling and being hurt," wrote one of my students in a report on Susan Sheehan's 1982 book, *Is There No Place on Earth for Me?*, a detailed account of several years in the life of a woman with schizophrenia.[1] "This is not something," the student continued, "someone would associate with a person who is mentally ill." This remarkable statement, which suggests that someone with a mental illness is not expected to have feelings or experience emotional hurt, is a perfect example of the kinds of inaccurate public expectations that constitute mental illness stigma.

According to *Webster's Dictionary*, stigma is "a mark of shame or discredit."[2] Erving Goffman reported on the word's origin in his seminal book on *Stigma*: Greeks introduced the word to refer to bodily signs designed to reveal the inferior moral and social status of individuals.[3] Slaves, criminals, and traitors had signs cut or burned into their bodies—quite literally they were branded—to signify that they were blemished and undesirable persons. Stigma was a characteristic that made clear that the possessors were to be looked down upon, avoided, and inferior.

Today, as Goffman noted, stigmas are usually not physical or bodily in nature. Personal, psychological, and social attributes are current stigmatizing characteristics. People are no longer physically branded; instead, they are societally labeled—as poor, criminal, homosexual, mentally ill, and so on. These labels influence public perceptions and behavior and lead to devaluation and denigration of those who are so labeled. Indeed, Stephen Ainlay, in writing about stigma as "the dilemma of difference," notes that the common feature of most definitions of stigma is that "all of them suggest in one way or another that stigma involves disvaluation of persons."[4] Whatever else they may be or have been, persons who possess a stigmatizing label become seen as less worthy of either respect or of inclusion in social intercourse.

The social effects of stigma have been underscored by a number of authors. Edward Jones and his colleagues, for example, referred to stigma as leading to "marked relationships," in which the responses of others are determined not by one's behaviors but by one's stigma.[5] The stigmatized enter interactions with others in a "one-down" position where they are already viewed unfavorably and it is unclear they can do anything to overcome the negative stereotypes their interaction partners may possess about them. This is especially true, Jones and Goffman both noted, when the stigmatized trait has the character of a "master status." That is, the stigmatized attribute becomes, in the eyes of others, the most important characteristic in judging and responding to the person; it thus pervades all social interactions. A person who has committed a crime and returns from prison, for example, may be indefinitely branded an "ex-convict," a label that implies a permanent lack of trustworthiness to many people. Regardless of the nature or circumstances of the past crime and despite whatever rehabilitation, learning, or character improvement may have occurred, potential roles as spouse, parent, employee, advocate, and so on, may continue to be limited by the distrust and dislike the "ex-convict" label brings. This pervasive and persistent undermining of social contact led Goffman to refer to stigma as "an attribute that is thoroughly discrediting" and to talk about stigma as producing "spoiled identity."[6]

Social scientists have also discussed stigma in terms of its likely impact on the thinking and behavior of the stigmatized individuals. One common observation is that stigma may become internalized whereby stigmatized individuals may come to share the same beliefs as the larger population and to view themselves in similarly disparaging ways. They may believe, like the rest of their culture, that people of a certain stigmatized status—say, welfare recipients—are inferior, flawed, unworthy, and so on; thus, should they find themselves in that same status, they will believe that they must have those unflattering characteristics as well. What follows becomes a kind of self-fulfilling prophecy: Believing that they are flawed, unworthy, and incompetent, stigmatized individuals may act in ineffective, unmotivated, or even pathological ways that then confirm the expectations that they and their society hold for them. Some scientists have even suggested that societal expectations place subtle pressure on stigmatized individuals to live up to (or perhaps down to) those role expectations.[7]

Most social scientists believe that these definitions and observations about stigma apply well to mental illness. Many, in fact, use mental illness as a prime example of the stigmatizing process: Those given psychiatric labels—either receiving direct professional diagnoses, seeking psychiatric treatment, or displaying behaviors connected in the public mind to mental illness—are thought to be "disvalued," to use Ainlay's term. They are seen as different from others—weak and flawed, less capable and less competent, with undesirable characteristics, such as dangerousness and poor grooming. Their opinions and feelings, presumed clouded by mental confusion, are not respected. Mental illness is seen as a prime example also of a trait with master status: it intrudes into all relationships; it casts doubt on the labeled person's ability to be a good parent, spouse, employee, or even citizen. Furthermore, those labeled as possessing the master trait of mental illness, it has been argued, accept the social definitions of their inferiority, feel ashamed and discouraged, and fulfill society's expectations by adopting the specified "mental patient" role.[8]

There is considerable anecdotal evidence to confirm that mental illness is a stigmatized condition. Take, for example, the long-standing devaluing of those with mental illnesses. People who showed psychiatric symptoms in thirteenth- and fourteenth-century Europe were often despised and punished as sinful and in league with devils and demons. In the early asylums of eighteenth-century Europe, psychiatric patients were held naked in chains in isolated cells with little heat or light based on the prevailing belief that mental illness rendered people less than human. They were believed to be like animals and hence oblivious to their treatment; the public was, in fact, invited to visit and view them (for a small fee) just as we visit zoos.[9] Similar attitudes were uncovered in the United States by Dorothea Dix, an early crusader for improved care of people with mental illnesses. Dix visited the prisons and poorhouses of nineteenth-century America and found people with mental illnesses housed in deplorable and inhumane conditions, "bound with galling chains, bowed beneath fetters and heavy iron balls attached to drag-chains, lacerated with ropes, scourged with rods and terrified beneath storms of execration and cruel blows."[10] Undoubtedly the most tragic example of this devaluing of people with mental illness was Nazi Germany's mass extermination of psychiatric hospital patients as possessing "life not worthy of life."[11]

Evidence that mental illness is a stigmatized condition comes not just from anecdote, however. Much social science research verifies the stigma of mental illness. First, numerous surveys of public attitudes toward mental illness have revealed strikingly negative views of psychiatric disorder and the people who suffer from it. In one early study done by Jum Nunnally in the late 1950s, four hundred individuals representative of the general population were asked to rate a number of different groups with respect to a list of bipolar adjectives (e.g., good-bad, safe-dangerous, predictable-unpredictable). The groups to be rated included "average man," "average woman," "psychiatrist," "child," "insane man," and "insane woman." Nunnally, finding that the adjectives most commonly associated with mental illness labels were decidedly unflattering, concluded that "old people and young people, highly educated people and people with little formal training—all tend to regard the mentally ill as relatively dangerous, dirty, unpredictable, and worthless."[12] Nunnally also compared the public's assessment of an "insane person" with its appraisal of a "leper" and found that expressed attitudes were much more negative toward the former; the "insane person" was viewed as more dangerous, insecure, unpredictable, bad, tense, and foolish than that historical symbol of social rejection, the "leper."[13]

As Nunnally's study and later studies have suggested, dangerousness is a key element of public beliefs about mental illness. Although the vast majority of those with mental illnesses, including severe illness such as schizophrenia, are not violent,[14] the public appears to believe otherwise, with their views shaped and reinforced by both fictional portrayals of psychotic killers and sensationalized news coverage of crimes committed by persons with mental illness.[15] A majority of California adults in a 1984 survey, for example, indicated beliefs that "schizophrenics" were more likely to commit violent crimes than other people.[16] Similarly, in a study of public knowledge of schizophrenia we conducted a number of years ago, approximately 35 percent of a sample composed of college students, community residents, and police officers indicated that they believed aggression and violence to be a common or very common symptom of that disorder.[17] In still another study involving telephone interviews of Utah residents, 38 percent of the five hundred interviewees reportedly agreed that "people with mental illness are more dangerous than the rest of society."[18] Even in a 1993 survey by *Parade* magazine, heralded as demonstrating improved attitudes toward mental illness, more than half the survey respondents agreed with the statement that "those with mental disorders are more likely to commit acts of violence."[19]

Evidence also suggests that the public views those with mental illness as characterologically, even morally, flawed. In a 1985 study, researchers presented adults from rural Tennessee with a written description of a person with prototypical paranoid schizophrenic symptoms and asked them various questions about their attitudes toward the person described. Most of the participants (75 percent) identified the man in the description as mentally ill, but more than half still indicated agreement with the statement, "This person should be viewed and treated as morally weak."[20] In the previously mentioned Utah study, 74 percent of the interviewees were reported to believe that "serious mental illness is caused by emotional weakness," 44 percent felt that "people with serious mental illness choose to be ill," and 35 percent even suggested that "serious mental illness is caused by sinful behavior."[21] And, as noted in the preface, 31 to 41 percent of respondents in a 1996 public opinion survey indicated beliefs that weakness in personal character contribute to depression and schizophrenia.[22]

Still other studies have shown that the tendency to attribute negative characteristics to those with psychiatric disorders is true for
health-care professionals as well as for the general public. John Fryer
and Leon Cohen, for example, asked employees at a Veterans Administration Medical Center to choose adjectives that described "patients
with medical problems" and "patients with psychiatric problems."
They found that patients labeled "psychiatric" were perceived by
hospital staff as overall less likeable than patients labeled "medical." In particular, psychiatric patients were characterized as more
apathetic, hostile, irritable, moody, argumentative, disorderly, im-
mature, impatient, irresponsible, selfish, dull, gloomy, and aloof than
the hypothetical medical patients; these characterizations led the
researchers to conclude that "professional caretakers share the general
public's stereotype of psychiatric patients as unpredictable, irresponsible, and socially undesirable."[23] Although caretaker expectations,
one might argue, are more informed by actual experience with
psychiatric patients than those of the general public (and thus more
"accurate"), this does not lessen the potential unfavorable consequences for individuals with labeled psychiatric conditions. Patients
with psychiatric disorders, Fryer and Cohen's results suggest, are likely
to be approached differently by professional caretakers from the start
of their interactions—with a more unfavorable set of preconceptions
and expectations—than are individuals with medical diagnoses.

Studies of people who believe they are interacting with individuals with a psychiatric treatment history likewise have revealed negative public attitudes. Amerigo Farina and Kenneth Ring conducted a
study in which research subjects were led to believe that the person
with whom they were working on a cooperative task had had prior
psychiatric hospitalization (even though that person, in fact, had had
no such hospitalization). Those who were told of the worker's former
patient status, as compared to those who were not told of any psychiatric history, tended to describe their coworker as less able to get
along with others, less able to understand others, less able to understand himself, and more unpredictable. They also tended to perceive
their coworker, inaccurately, as hindering performance on the joint
task.[24] In another study, research participants who listened to taped

interviews (actually identical scripted ones) reported disliking the interviewee more when they were told that the interviewee suffered from psychological maladjustment.[25]

In still another kind of study, the disparaging views of mental health professionals were revealed by having "normal" individuals pose as psychiatric patients. In one well-known study by David Rosenhan, eight "pseudopatients" applied for admission to a number of different psychiatric hospitals; they complained of auditory hallucinations (specifically, voices saying "empty," "hollow," and "thud") and used their own personal histories (except for disguising names and occupations). Somewhat to the surprise of the pseudopatients, who feared they would be quickly and embarrassingly exposed, all were admitted without question to the hospitals where they presented themselves. All pseudopatients also ceased reporting symptoms subsequent to their admission. Not only were they retained in the hospitals for stays ranging from seven to fifty-two days, but their in-hospital behavior was repeatedly seen as a reflection of their disorder, in line with Goffman's description of stigma as a master trait. When one pseudopatient approached staff with a question about his prescribed medication and began to write down the response (as part of the record he was keeping for the study), staff responded as if the inquiries were an anxious consequence of poor memory and replied: "You needn't write it. If you have trouble remembering, just ask me again." Pseudopatients worried that their recording of observations might reveal them as undercover researchers; instead, as later examination of entries in pseudopatients' charts revealed, their note-taking was merely interpreted as pathology and seen by staff as "engaging in writing behavior." Walking the halls out of boredom was interpreted as evidence of anxiety and agitation. Lining up early for lunch was seen as reflective of "the oral acquisitive nature of the syndrome." Once labeled mental patients, the individuals were viewed almost exclusively in terms of that label and thus subject to the negative expectations of the staff about their competence and motivations.[26]

Rosenhan's pseudopatients also experienced dramatic depersonalization and devaluing. Doctors and other staff accorded little respect to their questions or requests. For example, Rosenhan reported that the most typical response to legitimate questions about progress was "either a brief response to the question, offered while [the staff members] were 'on the move' and with head averted, or no response at all."[27] Such encounters, Rosenhan reported, frequently followed a script similar to this:

Pseudopatient: "Pardon me, Dr. X. could you tell me when I am eligible for grounds privileges?"

Physician: "Good morning, Dave. How are you today?" (Moves off without waiting for a response.)[28]

The notes of Rosenhan's pseudopatients revealed many other incidents, as well, when patients were treated as if they were either not there or certainly too unimportant to consider. This included observations of staff pointing to and discussing a patient in a group room as if he were not there and a nurse unbuttoning her blouse to adjust her brassiere in the presence of the entire ward. "Pseudopatients," Rosenhan noted, "had the sense that they were invisible, or at least unworthy of account."[29]

Examination of how mental illness is portrayed in the media reveals the consistent attribution of unfavorable characteristics to those with psychiatric disorder, as well. A 1981 evaluation of prime-time television—in which trained volunteers viewed and rated prime-time television programs over a one-month period—found that most characters labeled as mentally ill tended to be portrayed as lacking the social connections of jobs and families and tended to be best described by unfavorable adjectives such as "dangerous," "unpredictable," and "confused." Rarely were positive attributes, such as "honest," "loyal," or "friendly" associated with mental illness.[30] Nancy Signorelli, sampling twelve years of prime-time programming as part of George Gerbner's well-known Cultural Indicators Project, also found that mentally ill characters on television were less likely than other characters to have identifiable occupations and those who were employed were more likely to be shown as failures in those occupations.[31] Even more damning, mentally ill characters were consistently portrayed as violent and villainous. Despite recent research findings that show the rate of violence among non–substance-abusing persons with mental illness to be no greater than that of others in the neighborhoods in which they are living,[32] and despite repeated findings that the vast majority of people with mental illnesses (80 to 90 percent) are *not* violent,[33] television makes most of its mentally ill characters violent. George Gerbner and Nancy Signorelli, for instance, have reported that more than 70 percent of all mentally ill characters in prime-time drama and two-thirds of the mentally ill characters on daytime soap operas are depicted as violent.[34] More recently, Donald Diefenbach reported that crime in general and violent crime in particular were ten times greater for mentally ill characters on TV than for non–mentally ill characters and ten times greater than the actual rate of violence among those with mental illnesses in the United States population.[35] Moreover, Gerbner found that, when rating different groups of characters (e.g, Hispanic, African-American, elderly, female) as either heroes or villains, characters with mental illness were the only group more often portrayed as villains than heroes.[36]

Even in newspapers, there is a tendency to depict those with mental illnesses in unflattering ways. A 1991 study of the content of United Press International stories, for example, found that the majority of newspaper stories dealing with psychiatric patients involved the commission of violent crimes.[37] Another study arrived at a composite description of a person with mental illness derived from the typical stories about mental illness appearing in Canadian newspapers. According to that study, the typical person with mental illness depicted in newspapers is "dangerous, unpredictable, dependent, anxious, unsociable, unemployed, unproductive, and transient."[38] To the extent that these depictions reflect (and shape) public attitudes and expectations about mental illness, they confirm also the stigma that attaches to psychiatric disorder.

That the public attributes negative characteristics to those with psychiatric disorders is clear. So is the tendency of the public to make social rejection a consequence of mental illness. Numerous studies, in assessing mental illness stigma, have utilized "social distance" measures to establish the degree to which different types of individuals are accepted in different social situations. In these studies, people were asked to indicate their degree of comfort with mental illness in a variety of contexts. For example, one early social distance scale, used in a 1958 study by Charles Whatley, provided statements about the acceptability of different kinds of social interactions with former mental hospital patients and asked for agreement or disagreement with those statements. Whatley's results revealed that many people reported reluctance to accept former mental patients in any of the described roles. More than one-quarter (28 percent) of his two thousand participants agreed that "it would bother me to live near a person who had been in a mental hospital." Approximately one-third said that "I would not ride in a taxi driven by someone who had been in a mental hospital." One out of five even indicated that they agreed with the advice that "it is best not to associate with people who have been in mental hospitals."[39]

In another early study, Richard Lamy asked undergraduate students to choose between "the man who has been in a mental hospital" and "the man who has served a prison sentence" to complete a series of sentences. For example, "A lady having one single room to rent would less want to have for a roomer. . . . ", and "If they had to choose, most men would rather be. . . . " In most instances, the students chose the former convict over the former mental patient; this led Lamy to conclude that "the person who has had a mental hospitalization suffers a depreciation of social esteem in a wide range of social roles."[40] John Tringo also tried to assess the relative acceptability of people with mental illnesses. When he asked people to rate twenty-one different disability groups with respect to their social acceptability, he found mental illness to be rated at the very bottom, just below alcoholism, mental retardation, and being a former convict.[41] This is consistent with the 1968 findings of Zachary Gussow and George Tracy in which people rated various conditions and revealed their beliefs that the two most horrible things that can happen to someone are leprosy and insanity, consistent with Nunnally's findings that a man with leprosy is viewed more favorably than one with mental illness.[42]

Moreover, it is clear from some of these studies that rejection was in response to the person's label, not the symptomatic behavior. Consider the person described in the following way in one such study: "'Here is a description of a man. Imagine that he is a respectable person living in your neighborhood. He is happy and cheerful, has a good job and is fairly well satisfied with it. He is always busy and has quite a few friends who think he is easy to get along with most of the time. Within the next few months he plans to marry a nice young woman he is engaged to.'" This person, not surprisingly, was almost universally accepted by residents of a southern New England town participating in the study. All indicated willingness to work on a job with him, have him as a neighbor, or rent him a room; less than 2 percent were sufficiently protective that they would not allow him to marry their child. However, when the researcher added to this benign description the information that the man had once been in a mental hospital, the acceptance dropped markedly: fewer than half (40 percent) of the study participants expressed willingness to rent him a room and very few (only 17 percent) were not opposed to their daughter marrying him.[43] In another study, undergraduate students read vignettes that portrayed a person as having either cancer or schizophrenia and then were asked to rate the person with respect to a number of traits. The person identified as having schizophrenia was perceived as less desirable as a friend, less acceptable as a club member or neighbor, and less able to function in the community than the cancer patient despite the fact that the vignette descriptions (apart from the disorder suggested) were identical.[44]

Studies have established also that social rejection follows most forms of psychiatric treatment even without specific diagnostic labeling. Although social rejection scores were greatest when psychiatric hospitalization was the treatment disclosed, even having seen a psychiatrist as an outpatient generated reduced acceptance in social situations, as did, to decreasing degrees, having seen a physician or a member of the clergy.[45] As in other studies, display of symptomatic behaviors (via vignette descriptions) did not generate consistent rejection, but seeking help did. Having a mental illness label, even if it comes indirectly from having received treatment, is stigmatizing and leads to reduced social acceptance.

The mental illness label also has been shown to lead to discrimination. In a 1958 survey of two hundred employers, one out of every four reportedly stated that they would not hire a former mental patient, and many of those (40 percent) indicated they would hire the person only for a nondemanding, low-pressure job.[46] In another study, a researcher posed as a job applicant and obtained an interview at each of thirty-two manufacturing firms. Half the time he presented himself as having been traveling during the previous several months; in the other interviews, he indicated he had been in a psychiatric hospital. Despite identically solid resumes and background experience, which led to interview invitations, job offers were less likely when he disclosed previous psychiatric treatment, and job interviewers (secretly tape-recorded) were later judged to be less friendly toward the applicant who disclosed a psychiatric history.[47] In a similar study, job applicants to a Veteran's Administration hospital were evaluated by workers at the hospital. The applicant was less likely to get a job recommendation when he was presented as a former mental patient than when he was identified in his application as a former surgical patient.[48] In yet another study, directors of graduate medical training programs were asked to evaluate potential applicants. Applicants with a history of "psychological counseling" (but otherwise identical to other applicants) were judged less likely to be invited for an interview and less likely to be accepted into the training program.[49]

Discrimination in housing also was found to occur for those with mental illnesses. Female callers responding to rental ads were found to have more difficulty obtaining housing (being accepted as a tenant) when it was revealed that they were former mental hospital patients than when they did not report a psychiatric history. Often they were told that they were too late and that the apartment had already been rented, but, when another member of the research team called later to inquire about the apartment, no such discouragement was given.[50] Potential landlords, it was apparent, were responding on the basis of their negative beliefs about mental illness; they were responding not to any outrageous behavior of their applicants but to the stigmatizing label of mental illness.

The studies mentioned would seem to provide adequate evidence that stigma exists for mental illness. Most of these studies, however, are far from current; the majority of them were conducted in the 1960s and 1970s when research on mental illness stigma was probably at its peak. It is possible, certainly, that conditions have improved since the 1960s and 1970s and even 1980s and that public acceptance and understanding of mental illness has progressed. Although some more current studies (e.g., ones by Beldon & Russonello and by Bruce Link and his colleagues)[51] continue to provide evidence of mental illness stigma, there is clearly a need for more up-to-date research. One goal of the study described in this book was to provide such a current view of stigma.

Findings from previous studies of stigma, moreover, are limited in their ability to help us understand the specific experiences of people with mental illnesses. They allow us to predict what their experiences *may be* when they encounter negative attitudes in their communities. They do not, however, tell us clearly what the actual experiences of mental health consumers have been. Indeed, conspicuously absent from the above approaches to stigma is the person with the mental disorder who presumably carries stigma. Relatively few studies have sought information directly from mental health consumers, and even fewer have asked them about their experiences while interacting with the public.

In part, this dearth of direct study may be due to either the belief that one can accurately infer from the apparent attitudes of the public the probable experience of those with mental illnesses or to the desire for a more controlled (i.e., experimental or laboratory) methodology through which to gather data. Omission of consumer perspectives may reflect, as well, a desire not to intrude too deeply into the lives of people already sufficiently burdened (a view that, despite its good intentions, may be somewhat patronizing in its overprotectiveness). This relative neglect of first-hand data from mental health consumers may likewise be simply an extension of the general neglect of consumer input in all mental health efforts, including research—a neglect that may, in itself, reflect stigma and devaluation of those with psychiatric disorders. It may further reflect researchers' belief that input from those whose psychiatric disorders often impairs their perceptions and cognitions may be of little value. Researchers may be understandably concerned that consumers, because of their pathology, may not be able to accurately describe their experiences, although research evidence suggests that, given appropriately structured assessment tools, even those with considerable cognitive disorganization can provide reliable information about their lives.[52]

Direct input from consumers about their experiences can be of great value, however, and represents an important addition to other studies of stigma for several reasons. First, public attitudes, such as those assessed in other studies, do not directly translate into behavior; nor do studies of public attitudes reveal how those beliefs are conveyed. In addition, it is certainly possible that people learn to deny or disguise socially unacceptable beliefs on attitude surveys even though they retain them and act on them. Thus, knowing what people say about mental illness does not tell us precisely what those with mental illnesses experience in their encounters with others. In addition, even when negative public attitudes are expressed in behavior, it is not certain that they are perceived and reacted to by mental health consumers. The important and impactful specific events *in the daily lives* of the stigmatized individuals may not be exactly what others anticipate from public attitudes and analog studies. Furthermore, given that stigmatization has both overt and subtle manifestations, appreciation of the more subtle aspects may require the descriptions of those whose experiences have sensitized them. Even those posing as patients will not have had experiences fully comparable to those with real psychiatric disorders, for they surely knew that the attitudes they faced did not really apply to them, that they would soon be free of their fictitious psychiatric labels, and that they could return home after their experiences without anticipating lifetime recurrence.

Thus, direct input from stigmatized individuals with mental illness about their experiences can provide information simply unobtainable by other methodologies. It is unimaginable that we would try to understand racial and ethnic prejudices without hearing from racial and ethnic groups who have experienced it. Listening to African-Americans describe their discomfort at being watched more closely than Caucasian customers in mall stores or their awareness that others fearfully cross empty streets to avoid them helps us to appreciate the pervasiveness of prejudice and the less obvious ways it may be manifest. Full understanding of the specific ways mental health consumers encounter stigma and of the effects of these encounters on their own expectations, attitudes, and functioning is something that may be achieved only by input from consumers who have experienced real-life stigma.

In addition, the field of mental health care is beginning to appreciate the value and benefits of empowerment: when individuals and communities are strengthened they become better prepared to help themselves instead of relying on the interventions of presumably powerful professionals. Key elements of empowerment are the recognition of competencies inherent in individuals and communities, the acknowledgment of strengths they possess, and the communication of respect for those strengths. With regard to mental illnesses, this means viewing the individual as one who can make significant contributions to his/her own recovery, to others, and to the field of mental health in general, such as in the understanding of stigma. Empowerment, then, demands the greater inclusion of mental health consumers in decision making, in problem solving, and in research related to mental illness.

Listening to mental health consumers and providing opportunities for them to tell their unique stories is seen as an important strategy toward empowerment and self-esteem enhancement. Julian Rappaport, for example, has described the empowering (and therapeutic) aspects of shared stories. "The goals of empowerment," he has stated, "are enhanced when people discover, or create and give voice to, a collective narrative that sustains their own personal life story in positive ways."[53] Facilitating the telling of stories, then, is an important mechanism for giving consumers increased power over their lives. As Rappaport noted, "helping people to identify, create, and tell their own stories, individually and collectively, is an endeavor consistent with the development of empowerment."[54] Similarly, Charles Rapp and his colleagues assert clearly that "the adoption of an empowerment perspective requires that the consumer perspective be emphasized."[55] When consumers are excluded from input, the implicit stigmatizing message that their ideas are of little value undermines self-esteem. When consumers are not included in research on which interventions are based, furthermore, the result may be assistance that does not meet consumer needs. As Rapp and his coauthors have noted, "one of the reasons for the dominance of person-blaming interventions and research is that the people [whom clinicians] seek to help have not been judged to be important informants."[56]

When mental health consumers are excluded, when they are not asked about their disorders, the implicit message is that those in authority—the clinicians, the researchers, the policymakers—do not perceive their input as valuable. Even the perspectives they have gained from years of suffering are, it seems, worthless because they come from a person tainted with mental illness. In other words, such exclusion and neglect contribute to internalized stigma, while the empowerment of having one's ideas valued and sought may help to reduce the extent to which such internalized stigma occurs.

There are many reasons, then, to seek the input of mental health consumers about stigma. These reasons led us to undertake a nationwide study of consumers' experiences of stigma and discrimination and to write this book so that others could also learn of consumers' experiences. Consumer disclosures about their experiences are the substance of subsequent chapters.

3

Reaching

Consumers

Our research team had several goals in mind when we began preparing a study to learn more about consumer experiences of stigma and discrimination. We wanted to obtain information from as widespread a sample of consumers as possible. Most previous studies of stigma experiences among consumers tended to be limited to a particular organization and region. For example, one larger study of consumer experiences (noteworthy also because it was developed and executed by mental health consumers) was conducted as part of the California Well-Being Project.[1] The project involved 331 consumer respondents, all Californians. Another large study, completed in 1991 by Freedom From Fear—a patient-support group based in Staten Island, New York—surveyed 250 of its members.[2] A third large study, by Nancy Herman in 1993, included 146 former hospital patients from Southern Ontario, Canada.[3] We wanted to reach consumers in larger numbers in different settings across the nation: even more stories could be told, and the reported experiences would not be skewed by the biases of a specific group or the idiosyncrasies of a particular region or locale.

To accomplish this goal, we distributed our survey questionnaire in four different ways: First, the National Alliance for the Mentally Ill (NAMI) agreed to publish the questionnaire in the June 1996 issue of its newsletter, *The Advocate*, which circulates to more than 70,000 individuals and families affiliated with NAMI. Although most of these individuals are relatives of persons with mental illness, the published survey contained a request to pass it on to ill relatives and to any other consumers who might be interested in filling it out. Consumers were asked to return the surveys by mail to an address provided. Second, we approached NAMI's Consumer Council, composed of consumer representatives from across the country. Each of approximately thirty members of this council was given a starting packet of twenty-five survey questionnaires and asked to distribute them to consumers in organizations and programs in their home states whom they thought might be interested in providing us with input about their experiences. Stamped and addressed envelopes were provided for return of completed questionnaires, and additional questionnaire copies were provided upon request. Third, the questionnaire was placed on the internet via NAMI's website, and respondents could complete and return the survey electronically. Finally, some surveys came from miscellaneous sources. As individuals and organizations heard about the survey—from NAMI literature, from talks given by members of our research team, from conversations with others who had filled out the survey—they requested copies to circulate to consumers they knew who wished to contribute. Some photocopied the survey from the NAMI *Advocate* and distributed the copies to residential or day-treatment programs where they lived or worked; at least one person added the survey to his own internet site. In all cases, participants had the option of responding anonymously (i.e., names and addresses were not required).

Our goal of obtaining a large and diverse sample was largely met, as shown by the summary of participant characteristics in Appendix A. Altogether 1,388 completed questionnaires were received between 1 June 1996 and 1 January 1998; substantial numbers came from each of our distribution sources.[4] Approximately 64 percent (881) responded to the questionnaire through the NAMI *Advocate*.[5] Consumer Council distribution produced 268 survey responses (19 percent); internet posting of the survey led to 161 responses (12 percent); and a small number (74, or 5 percent) came from other unknown or miscellaneous sources.

As we had hoped, these participants came not from a single group or geographic area; instead, they came from all fifty states and the District of Columbia, as well as from Ireland, Wales, Australia, and

Canada—primarily via the internet. Most responses came individually, but some came in packets from a particular facility or program that had distributed and collected the survey. No one source or locale, however, was represented so strongly as to be able to significantly skew the results; no single state, city, or program contributed more than about 7 percent of the total. The greatest number of responses came from the states of California (95), Georgia (83), Minnesota (74), Pennsylvania (72), Ohio (66), and New York (61). The cities providing the most respondents were Milledgeville, Georgia (60), Jacksonville, Florida (35), Greenwood, South Carolina (33), Suitland, Maryland (26), Toledo, Ohio (26), and West Sacramento, California (22). The largest number of surveys received in any bulk mailing were from Unity Day Treatment (61) in Milledgeville, Georgia, and Beckman Center for Mental Health Services (33) in Greenwood, South Carolina (thus accounting for the large numbers from those two cities).

Respondents, moreover, came from small towns as much as from big cities: they represented more than 750 different zip code areas, including such places as: Gadsden (AL); Chuquiak (AK); Bullhead City (AZ); Conway (AR); Covina (CA); Westminster (CO); Tamarac (FL); Toccoa (GA); Post Falls (ID); Kankakee (IL); Farley (IA); Prairie Village (KS); Inkster (MI); Coon Rapids (MN); Florissant (MO); Rollingsford (NH); Jericho (NY); Lumberton (NC); Massillon (OH); Wewoka (OK); Wawa (PA); Chepachet (RI); Huron (SD); Cookville (TN); Lockhart (TX); Winooski (VT); Nine Mile Falls (WA); and Manitowac (WI).

Consumer respondents presented a diverse clinical picture as well, although not as fully diverse as would have been desirable. In particular, the majority of respondents (about two-thirds) had severe and persistent mental illnesses, with milder disorders less well-represented. The most frequent single diagnosis was bipolar disorder (25 percent), with schizophrenia (19 percent) and major depression (15 percent) also common.[6] A substantial proportion (14 percent) of the sample reported had been given multiple diagnoses—for example, depression and post traumatic stress disorder. An even greater percentage of respondents (18 percent) did not know or did not report their diagnoses. Diagnoses such as obsessive-compulsive disorder (0.7 percent) or other anxiety disorders (1.7 percent) were rarely reported. Consistent with the severe disorders experienced by most respondents, the vast majority (83 percent) reported that they had had at least one psychiatric hospitalization; the average number was six. The range was substantial, however; 17 percent reported they never had been hospitalized while 2 percent indicated that they had experienced thirty or more psychiatric hospitalizations. Thirteen individuals indicated that they had been hospitalized fifty or more times; the largest number was ninety-eight.

Disorders such as schizophrenia and depression are known to have their typical onset in adolescence and young adulthood; thus, it is unsurprising that the modal age at which respondents reported receiving their first diagnosis was eighteen. Again, there was a considerable range. About 7 percent of the respondents indicated that they had been diagnosed before age fifteen, and 5 percent reported that they had not received their first diagnosis until age forty-five or later. Several participants indicated that they had been diagnosed virtually from birth, while one person cited his/her age at first diagnosis as seventy-five.

Information provided about personal characteristics indicated a desired diversity, as well, albeit with some limitations. Respondents ranged in reported age from twelve to ninety-four, but only a very few were at those extremes. The average age was forty-two, and the bulk of respondents (87 percent) fell in the twenty-six to fifty-nine age range. Only about 6 percent were under twenty-five years of age, and 7 percent were sixty or above. This result is not surprising given the distribution sources closely tied to NAMI. As mentioned, NAMI is an organization that consists primarily of relatives—parents in particular—of people with severe mental illnesses. More than one-third of its members, according to a 1995 NAMI Member Survey, are age fifty-six or older; 62 percent are age forty-six and above.[7] Thus, many of the "children" to whom NAMI members might pass on the survey would be twenty-six and older. Indeed, members reported in the member survey that only about 7 percent of their relatives or friends with mental illness were age twenty-five or under.[8] Although our survey respondents' ages match NAMI demographics, they represent neither the population as a whole nor even the population of consumers. Clearly, the substantial population of younger people with mental illnesses remained unreached by our survey.

It is also true that minority populations were not well-represented in our survey. The vast majority of the respondents who reported racial identity were Caucasian, with notably few respondents who indicated that they were Hispanic (2 percent) or Asian (0.5 percent). As mental illnesses are, in general, equally common among all racial and ethnic groups, more minority representation would certainly be desirable. However, the representation in our sample of Caucasians (80 percent) and African-Americans (9 percent) is not markedly deviant from the general population, as shown in the 1997 United States census report, which indicated the population to be 75 percent Caucasian and 11 percent African-American.[9]

Given the average age of the responding consumers as forty-two and typical first diagnosis at age eighteen, these respondents have had many years of struggle with mental illness and ample opportunity to both experience stigma and react to it. Thus, they provided a good sample for describing stigma to us. As noted, however, the older age of respondents means that our findings may not fully represent people early in their experience as consumers. More information about the stigma experiences of younger consumers, who may be struggling with their first episode of mental illness and thus may experience stigma even more intensely, is needed.

Approximately 40 percent of those responding to the survey were male, and 56 percent were female. This slight gender skew may reflect the fact that some disorders represented (e.g., depression and manic-depression) occur more often among females. One might also attribute it to the possibility that females talk more readily about their problems and volunteer more readily for research surveys than do males; overrepresentation of females in research samples is common. Nevertheless, both males and females are well-represented in survey results, and it is unlikely that our findings are biased by the unique experiences of either gender. Most respondents were either never married (43 percent), divorced (23 percent), or widowed (2 percent); only about one in four (26 percent) were currently married. The percentage of married respondents is considerably below that of the general population (60 percent), while the percentage of those who have never married is substantially above that of the population at large (23 percent).[10] These differences probably reflect the fact that

mental illnesses take their toll on interpersonal and marital relationships, particularly the kinds of severe and early-onset disorders suffered by a large number of survey participants.

Respondents were diverse in their educational attainment as well.
Most tended to have had at least some college education (66 percent); 39 percent completed college, and 17 percent had completed
graduate or professional degrees. At the same time, the sample included a substantial number of people who had neither completed
(12 percent) nor gone beyond (17 percent) high school. An initial reaction to these data is that educational level is higher than might be
expected. The most common disorders experienced by survey participants, as noted previously, tend to have their onset in adolescence
or early adulthood—that is, in college years—and thus are likely to
interfere with the usual progression of schooling. Our survey respondents, then, may be more highly educated than the "typical" consumer with these disorders. However, I believe we need to make such
an interpretation cautiously and to consider the possibility that our
expectations are too low. The belief that those with serious, early-
onset psychiatric disorders cannot succeed in college and beyond may
reflect obsolete, inaccurate, and stigmatizing stereotypes, such as
those that are the focus of chapter 5.

The greatest number of consumers responding to our survey were
not currently working, although they had worked previously (46 percent). Four out of ten (40 percent) reported working either full-time
or part-time at the time of the survey. Many consumers reported
working in the health and mental health fields—as nurses, medical
assistants, dental hygienists, social workers, day-treatment providers, and psychiatric technicians. Others had as varied jobs as one
might expect in any general population. They were teachers, journalists, store clerks, dishwashers, carpenters, college instructors, ac-
countants, ministers, computer programmers and analysts, janitors,
legal secretaries, and telemarketers. Only 3 percent of respondents
reported never having been employed. That more than half of consumer participants were not employed (compared to about 5 to 6
percent of the general population) may,[11] again, reflect the disabling
nature of their disorders. It may also be a result of the operation of
stigma and discrimination that prevents those with psychiatric dis-

orders from gaining and maintaining employment, as described by our survey participants in chapter 6.

Most consumer respondents (61 percent) characterized themselves as living independently or semi-independently (for example, in supported community housing). About one in five reported living with parents. These results are consistent with what is known about the living situations of those with psychiatric disorders; most are not in institutions, but live in the community.[12] In addition, we had wanted not to restrict our sample of consumers only to those in or just discharged from psychiatric hospitals, as so many other stigma studies have done. The high proportion of respondents living independently and the 17 percent who had never been hospitalized suggests that we were reasonably successful. However, a sizeable population of mental health consumers exists in psychiatric hospitals, jails, homeless shelters, and on the streets.[13] That population was not reached by our survey; very few respondents were currently hospitalized (1 percent) or homeless (0.3 percent).

A second goal of our study was to find out about specific experiences of stigma rather than general perceptions or expectations about public attitudes and reactions. A number of previous studies with consumers have assessed primarily *the expectations* of mental health consumers, establishing that they anticipate being rejected and devalued. For example, Bruce Link, one of the most active researchers concerned with mental illness stigma, developed a twelve-item scale assessing consumer expectations that others will devalue or discriminate against a psychiatric patient once psychiatric history becomes known (for example, when a prospective job applicant has to explain the gaps in his resumé resulting from a period of hospitalization). The scale includes items such as: "Most employers will pass over the application of a former mental patient in favor of another applicant"; "most people think less of a person who has been in a mental hospital."[14] Similarly, Lisa Mansouri and David Dowell's (1989) assessment of consumers' experience of stigma asked for consumer judgment of how likely people were to do things such as "welcome you as a neighbor," "offer you a job if they had one available," "take you to lunch," and "accept you as their family's friend."[15]

Relatively few researchers have asked about the actual experiences of consumers; this absence opens them up to criticisms, like that of Walter Gove, that expectation of mistreatment is much greater than is warranted by actual experiences and that stigma, therefore, is less a problem than usually alleged.[16] Although fear of public reactions is important in its own right, regardless of its experiential basis, we wanted to know not just whether consumers *felt* stigmatized or *expected* to be poorly treated by others but what they had actually encountered in their interactions with their communities. Thus, our survey questionnaire cited specific types of situations and asked individuals how often they had experienced them. For example, on our survey we included specific types of incidents such as, "I have been treated as less competent by others when they learned I am a consumer"; "I have been shunned or avoided by others when it was revealed that I am a consumer." Survey respondents were asked to indicate whether they had experienced these events never, seldom, sometimes, often, or very often.

We also wanted to include experiences that were important to consumers but that might not have been touched upon in previous research. To accomplish this, we examined a large number of personal accounts of individuals with mental illnesses to see the kinds of things about which they expressed concerns. We reviewed the "First Person Accounts" the *Schizophrenia Bulletin* has published in each issue since 1979. We looked at autobiographical articles written by consumers in a special (1992) "Clients" issue of the *Journal of the California Alliance for the Mentally Ill*,[17] and we studied a similar set in the (1989) NAMI publication of *The Experiences of Patients and Families: First Person Accounts*.[18] Autobiographical books by people with mental illnesses—such as *An Unquiet Mind* by Kay Jamison,[19] *The Quiet Room* by Lori Schiller and Amanda Bennett,[20] *Undercurrents* by Martha Manning,[21] *Darkness Visible* by William Styron,[22] and *On the Edge of Darkness* by Kathy Cronkite[23]—also provided us with information about the personal experiences of people with mental illness. In addition, previous open-ended interview studies, such as those conducted by both Deborah Reidy and by Nancy Herman,[24] were used as a source of ideas for specific questions. Examining this literature we discovered, for example, that one commonly expressed concern—the frequent reminder to lower one's expectations in life—was seldom addressed in other stigma research. Furthermore, concerns about what we refer to as "indirect stigmatization"—seeing or hearing derogatory comments about mental illness even if they are not directed at the individual—were likewise common, but neglected in previous studies.

Finally, we consulted consumers directly in a pilot study; we prepared a preliminary questionnaire and asked for feedback from members of the NAMI Consumer Council as well as a consumer member of our research team about both the content and wording of the proposed instrument. We added several additional experiences based on input from these consumers. For example, Consumer Council members suggested that we should ask whether people had ever had their psychiatric history used against them in legal proceedings such as child custody or divorce and that we should ask about exclusion from volunteer activities as well as paid employment.

The resultant survey questionnaire involved three main sections. A "Stigma" section included nine questions about people's interpersonal experiences as consumers. Questions featured issues about specific treatment by others (e.g., being shunned or rejected), negative things seen or heard about mental illness (e.g., in mass media), and fears and behaviors related to disclosure of consumer status. As noted previously, respondents were asked to rate the extent of occurrence of each experience on a five-point scale from "never" to "very often." In addition, respondents were reminded to "base your answers on *your own personal experience*" rather than report what they thought might be true for others.

The second section, labeled "Discrimination," involved experiences of inappropriate denial of opportunity because of mental illness. This section included twelve items intended to explore the extent to which consumers had experienced discrimination in their lives (e.g., renting an apartment, getting a job, volunteering, getting a driver's license); these items also related to treatment in legal and law enforcement contexts as well as an avoidance of disclosure of consumer status on written applications. Again, items were rated on a five-point scale of frequency of occurrence from "never" to "very often."

It should be noted that the introduction to this section urged consumers to distinguish between lack of success (e.g., in getting a job) and discrimination. Instructions read:

> Please keep in mind that discrimination involves denial of opportunities *on grounds unrelated to your competencies* or level of functioning. If you are turned down for a job, for example, because your illness or your symptoms *are* interfering with your ability to fulfill the job requirements, that may not be discrimination. On the other hand, if you are turned down simply on the basis of your having had a mental illness or mental health treatment, without regard to your current abilities, that *would* be considered discrimination. Please keep this distinction in mind as you respond to the following items by circling the response which best fits *your* experience.

It is noteworthy also that each of these two sections had some items worded in a positive direction to reduce negative response bias. For example, one Stigma item, "I have been treated fairly by others who know I am a consumer," complemented one Discrimination item, "Co-workers or supervisors at work were supportive and accommodating when they learned I am a consumer."

A third section of the questionnaire provided consumers the opportunity to elaborate on their ratings ("Please use this space, if you wish, to explain or elaborate upon any of the responses to the previous questions.") or to tell us about experiences beyond those covered in previous sections ("Are there any other ways you have been treated differently—good *or* bad—once others learned you have had mental health treatment? Please explain.")[25]

The fourth section requested demographic and diagnostic information that would help us describe our group respondents: age, race, marital status, employment, diagnosis, living situation, and hospitalization history. Finally, the survey explained that we wished to interview some respondents and included a consent form to sign and return if the person were willing to be contacted for such an interview. A copy of the final survey can be found in Appendix B.

A fourth goal was to obtain qualitative, as well as quantitative, information so that we could not only learn the frequencies of occurrence of stigma experiences but also better understand specifically what happens to consumers. Requests for ratings of the frequency of occurrence of each questionnaire item provided a standardized quantitative means of describing consumer experiences. When someone said they have been rejected or shunned often, however, we wanted to know also the details of that shunning in order to achieve a better empathic understanding of the experience. What actually happened, when, and with whom? To obtain such information, we did two things: first, we invited all survey respondents to elaborate in writing on their responses to survey items; second, we conducted individual interviews with a selected sample of consumer respondents about the experiences they had cited. Interviews were conducted by telephone, tape recorded, and later transcribed verbatim. Trained doctoral students in clinical psychology did the interviews, which lasted between twenty-five and fifty minutes each. Selection procedures for those interviews are described below.

Because we lacked the resources to speak with all of the approximately 850 consumers who indicated they would be willing to be interviewed, we chose to interview about one hundred. However, we did want these to represent the larger group of respondents and used the following series of steps to select possible interviewees.

Each consumer respondent had an identification number assigned to him/her corresponding to the order in which the surveys were received. Because surveys were distributed through the different sources at different times (e.g., the survey appeared in the NAMI *Advocate* before it was posted on the internet) and thus responses from the different distribution sources tended to come in at different times, we chose a cohort method of selecting interviewees so that people from all different distribution sources might be included. Specifically, respondents were considered for interviews *within each cohort of one hundred*, with ten respondents interviewed from each cohort, when possible. Thus, we initially picked ten respondents at random (using a standard random number table) from the first one hundred, ten from the second one hundred, and so forth.

To be further eligible for interview, respondents identified by the cohort procedure had to have indicated on the written survey a willingness to be interviewed *and* to have indicated at least two stigma experiences and two discrimination experiences having occurred often or very often in their lives (i.e., they had to have stigma and discrimination experiences to tell us about). Eligible respondents in the first cohort of one hundred were contacted until ten persons had been interviewed from that cohort. Then respondents from the second (and then third and then fourth, etc.) group of one hundred were contacted using the same procedure until a maximum of ten had been interviewed from each cohort. Occasionally, ten interviews could not be obtained from a 100–respondent cohort; an additional eight needed interviewees were then obtained from the 1001–1388-respondent cohort.

Occasionally, individuals who had indicated a willingness to be interviewed on the written survey either changed their minds or expressed reservations when we contacted them for the interview. Furthermore, some selected respondents who indicated willingness to be interviewed neglected to provide phone numbers for contact; still others could not be reached despite repeated calls. Thus, many more individuals were selected and called than were actually interviewed. It also turned out that cohort quotas were easier to obtain among earlier respondents than later ones. For example, ten interviews were accomplished from the first sixty-five respondents identified by random number in the initial (1–100) cohort, but only four interviews could be obtained from the entire 800–900-respondent cohort. It was the impression of interviewers that later respondents were somewhat less well-functioning than those who were motivated and organized enough to respond right away. It was also true that more of our later responses came in group rather than individual mailings. Some day-treatment and group-home programs, perhaps as a result of Consumer Council members' urging, apparently distributed survey questions to their members, collected them, and mailed them in bulk; these tended to arrive later than the surveys filled out individually from the NAMI *Advocate*. It may be true, then, that later respondents were somewhat less recovered (still in treatment programs) than earlier respondents (and, not having individual or family telephones, harder to contact). These possibilities provide further support for our cohort approach by allowing us to include early (perhaps more well-functioning) respondents as well as later (perhaps less well-organized) respondents as interviewees.

For the most part, we successfully obtained a group of interviewees that was similar to our overall consumer sample and reasonably diverse, as shown in the summary of interviewee characteristics in Appendix C. Interviewees, for example, came from forty different states and ninety-eight different zip code areas. The largest number of interviewees who came even from the same state was seven (California) with Pennsylvania and Texas contributing the next most (six). Interviewees came from distribution sources in proportions roughly comparable to those of the overall survey sample: the majority (74 percent) responded to the NAMI *Advocate* (vs. 64 percent of the total sample), 17 percent (vs. 19 percent) responded through Consumer Council distribution, and 9 percent responded (vs. 12 percent) via the internet. As with the overall sample, interviewees were predominantly Caucasian (84 percent vs. 80 percent of the total sample) and similar in age (average = 42.7) to those in the larger sample (average = 41.9).

In terms of clinical picture, interviewees were again quite similar to those in the overall survey group. The most common diagnoses were bipolar disorder (28 percent for interviewees, 25 percent for the total sample), schizophrenia (17 percent and 18 percent), and major depression (16 percent and 15 percent). The only clear diagnostic difference between the interview group and the overall sample was in the much greater frequency of multiple diagnoses among the interviewees (29 percent vs. 14 percent). As with the full sample, the greatest number of interviewees had been hospitalized between six and twenty times, although their average number of hospitalizations (7.2) was slightly higher than that of the full sample (5.7).[26] Given these many similarities, we have reasonable confidence that our interviewees are representative of the larger number of consumers who responded to our initial survey.

A final goal was to go beyond the stigma experiences themselves and look also at consumer reactions to those experiences. We wanted to understand how such experiences affected the individual, in both short and long terms. We desired also to learn about how consumers coped with stigmatizing experiences, especially about successful coping. Information about successful coping with negative experiences, we believed, might be particularly useful to both consumers and mental health professionals. Along these same lines, we also wanted to take advantage of the possible wisdom gained by consumers who had lived with and learned from stigma and to find out what recommendations they might have about how stigma could best be countered and reduced. We used our follow-up interviews to obtain this information. Specifically, the interview included questions such as:

What have you done to deal with the stigma of mental illness?

What strategies have been helpful to you?

What do you think needs to be done to reduce the stigma of mental illness?

If there was one message you could give people about mental illness, one request you could make to them, what would it be?

One thing that was immediately obvious in the response of consumers was their desire to be heard. Not only did a large number of consumers take the time to complete and return survey questionnaires, but they did so eagerly. More than four hundred responses were received within the first two weeks following the appearance of the survey in the NAMI *Advocate*. Almost one-third (31 percent) of our respondents took additional time to elaborate on their responses by writing in the space provided for elaboration, adding information on the back of the questionnaire, and/or appending additional pages. Some also sent newspaper or newsletter articles they had written previously about their experiences; one even sent a copy of his published book. Another enclosed a photograph to demonstrate that "contrary to popular public belief we consumers are not all drooling, babbling to ourselves or carrying semi-automatics ready to mow the world down."

In addition, many respondents added notes thanking us for conducting the survey and for showing an interest in consumers' experiences. One respondent, for example, wrote: "Thanks for giving me the opportunity to speak about stigma issues from a consumer viewpoint." Another wished: "God speed to anyone who is working on mental health issues. . . . We appreciate it and it is needed in America." Still another added: "Nobody really understands what it is like to suffer a mental disorder unless they have one themselves. And I don't think this is an easy situation to resolve. I hope some good comes out of this survey."

Consumers' eagerness to provide input was revealed also in their responses to our survey question about whether they would be willing to be interviewed as a later part of the study. Despite our concerns that—in part because of the stigma of mental illness—consumers would prefer to remain anonymous and be reluctant to be interviewed and tape-recorded, almost two-thirds of our respondents provided their names and phone numbers and indicated that they would be willing to be interviewed for the study. More than just willing to be interviewed, some asserted that they wanted very much to be interviewed and have the opportunity to further tell their stories. One respondent stated:

> I really wish I could be interviewed by you guys. Yes I have a lot to tell you about things because of mental illness. . . . If you want to interview me person to person I'll be real happy to talk because I have pain locked in my heart from these hospitalizations until I thought I'll never get to express my feelings. So yes I am asking you to interview me. . . . So please if you must give me a chance to express my feelings and the rejection I've had to face because of being an ill patient. O.K. Thank you for wanting to care about us mentally ill people.

Many consumers, eager to participate in the study as a means to assist others similarly affected, liked the idea of being able to do something that might assist other consumers. They welcomed the chance to take an active, helping role contrary to the passive role of victim of mental illness and stigma. As one person indicated: "I've been through hell and am willing to talk about it to anyone who will listen. I want people to understand mental illness . . . and to remove stigma. If there is anything I can do to accomplish this, please let me know." Another echoed these thoughts: "Please call me if you would like to talk to me about anything. I would be most happy to help in any way I can!"

The rapidity, eagerness, and gratitude apparent in consumer responses were also, no doubt, a by-product of the previously noted neglect of consumer perspectives. Although arguably consumers hold the greatest stake in improving public understanding and treatment of mental illnesses and know the most about those illnesses, their impacts, and consumers' needs, the consumers themselves have historically been excluded from research and treatment planning. It was clear from the comments of consumer respondents that they appreciated this survey as a rare and long overdue chance to be heard. On an even more personal and emotional level, implicit in their remarks was the perception of a therapeutic opportunity to unburden themselves about the troubling ways they have been perceived and treated, something that, even in the course of their ongoing treatment (with its typical focus on medication management, emotional control, practical problem solving, etc.), they rarely have a chance to discuss. "Thanks for giving me the opportunity to speak about stigma issues from a consumer perspective," wrote one respondent. "I am grateful for a chance to share my story where it will be heard," said another. And still a third wrote: "I am delighted that you have given me the opportunity to address the issue of stigma, for as you can imagine, it is never far from my mind."

Finally, we noticed an implicit sense of appreciation that their input was being valued and respected and that there was someone, in addition to other consumers or their families, who wanted to know about their experiences. Many respondents seemed excited that someone of professional stature—a researcher, a mental health professional, a university professor—would recognize their expertise on the issue of stigma and value their input enough to seek it out from across the country. As one consumer wrote at the top of his/her completed survey: "I just want you to know first of all that I'm thankful that somebody cares."

4

Isolation and

Rejection

When people are stricken by whatever strain of influenza is making its seasonal rounds, and its symptoms send them to bed with fevers, chills, and nausea, it is usual for their friends, relatives, and coworkers to express their sympathy. Some stalwart friends may even brave contagion to visit with hot soup and good wishes. Should acquaintances be afflicted with something more serious, perhaps even something that requires them to go to a hospital—a heart attack or cancer, for example—others may be even more solicitous. They are likely to inquire of the sick individuals' families about their health, visit them at the hospital, and send cards and flowers to try to cheer them up. When the patients are better and return to work or social activities, someone is sure to communicate pleasure that they are back on their feet, and there will be little hesitation about welcoming them back into their previous circle of friends and colleagues.

A far different scenario emerges if the affliction suffered happens to be a mental illness. Rather than receiving an outpouring of sympathy and support, according to the consumers in our survey, those with mental illnesses are more likely to experience avoidance and rejection. One of the most common experiences reported by mental health consumers in our survey was being shunned and rejected by others. Of our respondents 61 percent indicated that they had at least sometimes been shunned or avoided by others when it was revealed that they were mental health consumers. More than one-quarter

(26 percent) said this had happened to them often or very often. "What really hurts," summarized one consumer, "is when people shy away from you like you have a plague."

Such rejection is, of course, the predicted response, given the previous research on public attitudes. The general population's negative appraisals of people labeled as psychiatric patients apparently translate into avoiding such individuals. Consumer reports of frequent shunning are also consistent with previous smaller surveys of consumer experience. In a 1989 study designed and conducted by mental health consumers, for example, 331 mental health consumers in California either received a structured interview or filled out questionnaires about a variety of issues. Of the respondents, 41 percent reported being treated "differently" by others when their status as psychiatric patients became known, while fewer than half (41 percent) were able to say that they felt accepted in social situations most of the time.[1] Similarly, a 1997 study by Bruce Link and his colleagues, involving eighty-four men with mental illness and substance abuse problems, found that 37 percent of the respondents to a stigma survey reported having been avoided by others.[2]

Thus, it is not at all surprising that many consumers in our survey reported being shunned and avoided by others. Their reports, however, went beyond mere rating of significant rejection, and, in their interviews and written comments, consumers revealed the variety of ways and circumstances in which such shunning occurs—as well as the variety of sources from which it came.

Sometimes shunning was relatively subtle, a probably unintentional product of discomfort and uncertainty on the part of others when they learned they were dealing with a person with mental illness. As shown in a 1991 Louis Harris public opinion poll, people are often uncomfortable around someone with a disability. In fact, of the disabilities covered in the Harris poll (mental retardation, hearing impairment, visual impairment, senility, wheelchair use, facial disfigurement, and mental illness), wheelchair confinement was the only disability with which the majority of people said they would feel comfortable. The most commonly described discomfort was feeling awkward and embarrassed: people do not know what to do or say in the presence of a person with a disability. Moreover, the Harris poll showed that discomfort is particularly pronounced with mental illness; only 19 percent of survey respondents indicated that they were very comfortable with a person with mental illness, as opposed to 39 percent who reported being very comfortable with people who are deaf and 59 percent with people who are in wheelchairs. More poll respondents were comfortable with people who are facially disfigured (28 percent) than with people who have mental illness. "From the public's perspective," the Harris poll concluded, "mental illness is the most disturbing form of disability."[3]

The public's discomfort with mental illness was communicated to consumers in many ways—looks and gestures, abbreviated conversations, avoidant behavior. "Most don't know what to say and feel uncomfortable and nervous," noted one respondent to our survey. "They look at me with wide eyes and say nothing, or quickly end the conversation." "I felt like there was just more of a reluctance to interact with me," observed another, "that people kind of shied away from me and didn't talk to me as they did prior to when all that happened. . . . When I go to interact with somebody, I feel like they really want to keep the conversation as brief as possible, and that they're uncomfortable with the conversations. And that people that ordinarily, prior to [when] . . . this whole thing came up, we could talk about anything." "When I have mentioned that I have a mental illness," noted another, "I have seen people obviously taken aback and then it seems like the end of the conversation. . . . It's the way they look. I can see they feel discomfort." A fourth said simply, "People with little or no knowledge of mental health issues sometimes back away from me." One person described a particularly memorable interaction when others knew of her psychiatric disorder: "Out of a group of eleven in a restaurant, the girl sitting beside me kept pulling her chair away, scooting to the side as if touching me would contaminate her. I at first thought this may be 'all in my head.' I tapped her on the shoulder and she jumped and practically bit my head off, asking what I wanted. . . . She made it very plain that she would rather not talk with me because she 'just wasn't sure of me.'"

A key element of the public's discomfort around mental illness, as revealed in previous research on public attitudes, is the fear that mental illness renders people violent and dangerous. When someone learns that a coworker or neighbor has had a psychiatric disorder, they begin to imagine that this person could go berserk at any time and act violently toward them; it is not surprising that this misconception creates discomfort and avoidance. Consumers, sensitive to such discomfort, were well aware of being feared by others. One consumer, for example, observed: "There are people if I tell them I suffer from mental illness they think I will take their lives just like Jeffery Dahmer." "If you mention that you are going to see a psychiatrist, people get kind of panicky," said an interviewee. "They think maybe you need to be locked up or that you're going to attack them." "I could say people shy away because they are afraid of me," wrote another, "afraid I might go berserk or behave badly and embarrass them." Some consumers even came to accept such frightened withdrawal as almost unavoidable: "My experience is that most . . . people react with fear and draw assumptions based on the mere elaboration that I have undergone mental stress and subsequent treatment. This reaction seems almost instinctive to most individuals."

The fearful avoidance consumers experienced was, again, both subtle and overt. One woman described how explicit concerns about her possible dangerousness have put a strain on family relationships: "In 1983, I met my husband-to-be. His mother (an R.N.) was *outraged* that he would consider dating a woman on meds for depression! She told him things like I could turn psychopathic at any moment. It's amazing that a trained health worker could be so ignorant about depression. We've been married twelve years, and she continues to hold this against me. It has been very stressful for the whole family." Another consumer explained: "I've seen some people kinda shy away from my work area because they're afraid of being around the people with, quote unquote, certain disabilities. They would, instead of walking past a work area to their desk, they'd walk around a work area, take a slightly longer route to get to their desk because . . . telling by their body language, they're afraid of the nuts at one end of the office." Fearful suspicion of mental health consumers also was conveyed, noted this same consumer, when the luxury hotel at which a meeting of consumer advocates was being held "asked for extra security people to come in because of the people with mental illness."

Several people mentioned how fears of mental illness were manifest in their community's sudden concern about the children with whom they might have contact. "Everything would be fine within the community," explained one woman, "until I would have an episode. . . . Then no one would talk to me or allow their children to play with my children." Another observed: "When I moved to [this town] people were very nice, [but] when I had a reoccurrence of depression and several hospitalizations, a few would no longer let their children come over to play. I wish I had not been so honest about being in a psych hospital." A third reported: "I have worked as a teacher. When parents found out I was in treatment and hospitalized for a medication balance, two children were removed from my classroom because their parents did not want their children to be around a person like that." Another said similarly: "I am an elementary school teacher, and parents, once learning I am manic-depressive, would request their children not be placed in my class or would simply request someone else." "People are fearful to have me around their children," said yet one more respondent, adding also that people even seemed to believe "that I should not be ALLOWED to raise my own."

From these consumer reports it was clear that people responded to their fears and discomfort by attempting to keep consumers at a distance or by avoiding them altogether. What consumer descriptions indicated, furthermore, is that such avoidance came from not only strangers or casual acquaintances but also those who knew them well—people from whom they had expected better. "I have been shunned by people who had known me for years," one person stated simply. Sometimes those were people whom the consumer had considered "friends." Although the majority (83 percent) of respondents agreed with the statement that "friends who learned I am a consumer have been supportive and understanding," the occurrence of damaged or lost friendships was nevertheless mentioned many times by the people who shared their experiences with us. One in six (16 percent) indicated that friends had seldom or never been supportive.

Sometimes the problem was that friends failed to provide support in time of psychiatric crisis. "I was employed as a counselor," said one interviewee, "and I had been hospitalized. . . . People who I thought were friends didn't call or check up on me or anything. . . .

That was hard for me to deal with, especially since I was feeling so down about myself anyway. It was very upsetting." "The thing that is most devastating for people that are mentally ill," observed another, "is that they are completely ostracized by their friends. . . . I think you're really hurt by friends that you have known all your life. And, all of a sudden, the phone quits ringing and they quit coming to the house. And, by glory, that's when you need them to come to the house and talk to you." Still another reported: "There's a pretty close group of people that I work with . . . and they've all known me for a very long time. Of those people, [there were] only three that had bothered to call me when I was in the hospital just to talk with me or [visited and] talked with me. . . . I was angry, hurt."

In other instances, disclosure of a psychiatric disorder impaired or ended the relationships altogether. One man who worked as a firefighter recounted how "once I entered the hospital in 1990, the firefighters, friends of mine, had little to do with me. . . . Christmas cards that we used to exchange in the past don't happen any more. Telephone calls are few and far between. If I make a phone call and leave a message, messages aren't returned." "I had one gal that I worked with and we were pretty close together," said one of our interviewees. "We worked together, same shift. And I told her that I had had a nervous breakdown, and I had been mentally ill for about three years. And after that she just kinda, we couldn't do anything together because she would find an excuse. We couldn't do anything together because she had something to do." This type of experience was repeatedly described by our interviewees: "I told my friend S. [about my mental illness], and I never heard from her again." "I still share friendships with only three of my friends out of many that I had prior to my diagnosis." "I have had people when I got sick and have gone for treatment that dropped me as a friend." "I had one friend that I had been friends with for over twenty years. When she found out that myself and my daughter have this problem, it was just as if she turned off a light switch. She wasn't calling. She wasn't coming over. She wouldn't go anywhere with me."

Dating and romantic relationships were also reportedly harmed by revelation of mental illness. "Several 'girlfriends' who had great affection for me have made a literal about-face after I revealed I was schizophrenic," reported one consumer. "I have had difficulty in keeping sexual partners once they find out that I'm a consumer," reported another. A third explained: "I can think of three instances where I was pretty much devastated by getting in a close relationship with a member of the opposite sex and then, at some point, when I felt comfortable, revealing to this person that I had a problem with mental illness. And in each of these three instances, the person quickly rejected me and ended the relationship." "I was dating a man one time," explained still another, "and he told me that he was afraid. He really loved me, but he was afraid to marry me because he thought I might end up in a mental institution. And I thought that was one of the cruelest things I'd ever been told."

A few consumers commented also on the difficulty of starting new relationships with a psychiatric history to overcome. Just as old friends withdrew, potential new friends were scared away by knowledge of the person's mental illness. This was especially true for dating and romantic relationships. "People who might have dated me backed off," noted one consumer. "If you try to [date] somebody outside of the [mental health] system," observed another, "they're frightened by what they've heard and what they think the illness is. They usually scare off." As Deborah Reidy pointed out in her study of consumer experiences, titled "Stigma is Social Death," the result of telling is that consumers' social circles become limited to mental health facilities where they meet (and sometimes marry) other consumers.[4]

Such isolation is painful, particularly when it comes at a time—recovering from a serious illness—when social support is especially needed. "At work, they may say good morning or hi," explained one of our survey respondents, "but I am never asked to social gatherings outside of work. People think I am defective or that I may become violent or something. So they don't even consider me a person because they don't understand 'people like us' and even seem scared of me, even though I have never been violent around them, only a good worker with no threat to them whatsoever. I do have feelings, and it hurts to be treated as a nonperson." The exclusion from activities that may be pleasurable and could help to ease the burden of emotional illness was likewise a source of pain for consumers. One consumer, for example, described this sequence of events: "[On one occasion] I was asked to go to Lexington, Kentucky, a wonderful town I went to a great deal during college years. After twelve years I was getting to go back, and see the new bookstore, and visit the Disney store. I saved my money and planned, excited each day about going. [Then my friend] asked her other friends to go . . . and 'forgot' to tell me. I knew [I was not invited] so I called and said I couldn't go. All the while my heart was shattered at not getting to go because I was different and made others uncomfortable. Thanks to the Risperadol [a treatment medication], I did it with polish . . . but it didn't ease the pain or dry the tears I shed at being labeled."

It was particularly painful also when the rejection and avoidance came from those to whom one usually turns for support and understanding. Some consumers, for example, were surprised and hurt by lack of support from their religious communities: "My church people have basically been my church family," said one devout churchgoer. "[But] when I came back [from a psychiatric hospitalization], everybody was really cold towards me . . . ignoring me, almost looking over me like I'm not there." "My deepest pain is with church families," wrote another saddened consumer. "It has happened to me twice in two states. . . . When I've been ill, the backs of church families were towards me. The way most people discriminate is by their silence and disappearance in your life. It doesn't matter that I've been an active church member and tithed hundreds of dollars a month." "I told the minister and a woman's outreach worker from church (who wondered if it was okay to take me to a restaurant for coffee) about it and they disappeared," explained still another consumer. "They knew I was about to have surgery for cervical cancer but never stopped by the hospital or called me. I never heard from them again." Even the pastor of a church revealed a tale of hurt and disappointment:

In August 1990, I had just begun my sixth year in a growing pastorate. Although I was struggling with depression. . . . I said little to members during my pastorate. I had often heard them make fun of two previous pastors who had had mental breakdowns while serving them as their pastor. I broke in August 1990. My elders quickly agreed to abandon me and tell the congregation not to call or visit me. . . . I spent three months being treated as a leper by a congregation I had given my everything to. They wrote me a dismissal letter and . . . proceeded to hire another pastor. Even when I came out of the hospital, I was told not to attend special services going on being led by my own personal friends I had invited. I was never invited back to say goodbye.

The general public whose negative attitudes toward mental illness fuel rejection and avoidance appeared to include family members as well. Some families treated mental illness—and their ill members—as a source of shame and embarrassment. "I grew up in a family that people going to the hospital, they just totally kept it quiet," explained a woman whose depressive disorder led her to treatment. "We don't talk about that. It was like they were so embarrassed that they would just deny that it ever happened. And it was real hard because my mother would never visit me when I was in the hospital. It's just like you don't exist when you're in there, and that was just real hard because I felt rejected and abandoned." Numerous other consumers reported similar experiences: "My own sister has publicly said she finds it an embarrassment . . . and at times she wishes I 'had been born normal.'" "My family seldom visited me in the hospital because they were ashamed of me and felt my being sick made them look bad." "My family members were extremely non-supportive. . . . They were just so ashamed. And they made me more ashamed of myself."

Family rejection was, at times, even more severe, as when consumers found themselves completely cut off from their families when they became ill. "My husband's family completely dropped us," reported one woman. "They stopped sending me Christmas cards, stopped sending me birthday cards, stopped coming here. They live an hour and a half away. They haven't been to visit for at least ten years." Another reported that: "My daughters haven't talked to me in almost two years. They're ashamed and disgusted that I can't hold a job or at times even go out in public. The oldest acts like I'm dangerous, so she wouldn't let me see her daughter. I haven't seen my granddaughter in almost two years. She doesn't know me any more." A third explained that: "My kids stay away the most. . . . They completely stay away," adding that "the most recent thing that's really hurt is my oldest son finally gave me a grandchild, but him and his wife separated and divorced and she has put in the divorce papers that I am never to be alone with my grandson because of my condition." Still another distraught parent had this story to tell:

> I have a twenty-seven-year-old son who will not speak to me because I'm mentally ill. He's a successful young man and he doesn't want the stigma of both poverty—because I was forced to accept [social security]—and someone that's been labeled as mentally ill. It's a deterrent to his future opportunity. . . . I found a missing persons service to find him, wrote him letters, and he refuses to contact me. And the feedback I got from the missing persons service was he does not want to be associated with a mentally ill mother.

The rejection that consumers reported sometimes took forms other than simple avoidance or exclusion. For example, consumers sometimes felt blamed for their illnesses and for the burdens they were creating for others. As one respondent described it: "The ongoing theme is that it is your fault, *you* are wrecking other people's lives by your illness, and you should apologize for it. People often look at me with a cruel look as though I have wronged them, sometimes merely because I admitted to them I had a mental illness." This person also recounted how "one person who was present during my first psychotic break, and who has been kept abreast of my situation throughout my illness was very vocal in making comments like 'How dare she do such a thing to her parents!'"

Because mental illness is an invisible disability—that is, one that is not outwardly apparent like many physical disabilities—it was sometimes difficult for others to understand why the consumer was not functioning better. They did not understand why the person was not employed full-time or why he or she should be receiving social security or other disability support. "I have two friends who get disability," explained one of our respondents, "and to everyone else . . . they are robbing the government or whoever for a free ride." Convinced that those with invisible mental disabilities are not truly disabled, people then tend to interpret consumers' nonproductivity as signs of character or moral weaknesses, consistent with the findings of the studies reviewed in chapter 2. Such views seemed to serve as a source of experienced rejection by many in our survey.

Consumers described, for example, how others refused to believe that their illnesses were "real"; instead, others saw consumers' problems as failures of motivation, effort, or will, an assessment that leads to rejection of the consumer as lazy, weak, willful, or self-indulgent. "There are just a few people," reported one woman, "who will say real loud in front of people if I am outside, say 'Well, there is somebody that don't want to work for a living and just wants to sit back and draw social security by pretending to have a problem.'" "My father tells everyone that will listen," lamented another, "that his daughter is a lazy, fat slut who does nothing but sit in front of the TV and EAT!" A third reported that "my late mother would call my sister (who has the same mental illnesses as me) and me lazy, senseless, stupid, etc." A fourth person noted similar family reactions: "The family members feel that I'm just doing this to get out of the housework and there's no excuse for me being like this. . . . And tell my husband that, why doesn't he kick my hind end and make me do what I'm supposed to do." Yet another respondent reported: "I remember one friend specifically saying, 'Well, why do you have to have this problem. . . . There was some perception that I was lazy . . . that I wasn't really trying to do anything in my life."

An assessment of consumers as lacking in some socially disapproved way was perceived also in the advice reported by many consumers: observers often insisted that the consumers would not have the problems attributed to their mental illnesses if only they were more resolute, more motivated, or more optimistic in their outlook. "From the time of onset [of my disorder], I had always been frustrated and angry because I couldn't get anyone to believe me," explained one of our interviewees. "It's like nobody ever wanted to believe that it was real. It was always presented to me like it was a choice. 'Well, you don't have to be nuts. You don't have to be depressed. Just change your mind.'" "I've heard many people tell me (through the years) that I *could be happy* if I chose to be," reported a sufferer from bipolar disorder, "and that if I made up my mind I could do without 'those pills'—'you just think you need them.'" Medication, in fact, was particularly singled out as a source of criticism and rejection from others; the need for continued medication apparently signals weakness and dependence—even addiction. "I have run across people who accept the fact that I have a mental illness," wrote a consumer, "but discriminate against me if they know I take medication. They have the feeling that they don't even take an aspirin for a headache and if I got off my meds I'd be a whole lot better. . . . My friends still ask 'Why do you have to take pills?' I feel this ignorance is partly due to the 'war on drugs' and I am a 'druggie' and no better than addicts who smoke dope or are hooked on heroin." Said another: "[People] want to know why you're taking the medication, and, if you mention it's for depression or something like that, they say things like, 'Well you could get along without that medication if you made up your mind to. The only reason you're depressed is because you don't try to be happy. You can get yourself out of the depression if you make up your mind to be happy." Still another reported: "The neighbor down the street from us . . . I told her that I'm taking medication for [depression] and she said that I need to learn how to cheer myself up."

A Catch-22 emerges in some reports by several consumers: If people are reasonably successful in coping with their psychiatric disorders and in finding treatments that effectively control symptoms, then they are even more vulnerable to accusations that their disability is not real and that their own character flaws underlie any problems they experience. "There are some people," observed a respondent, "who think that those of us with mental illness/brain disease should or will behave in a bizarre fashion or we are not truly ill. . . . [One woman] indicated that she had observed me when I was out and I didn't show any signs of bizarre behavior, so I must be faking my disability. . . . [Others] have made their own diagnosis of me, and thanks to my medicine controlling my psychotic episodes they have dubbed me a drain on the government, a burden who lives off my parents."

Views of mental illness as a religious failure, spiritual weakness, or sin were encountered as well. "I've had a number of comments," reported one interviewee, "that the devil is doing this to me, and I need to rebuke the devil. . . . And then I had another woman [tell] me that God doesn't have anything to do with sickness because God is a loving God and that I obviously had done something wrong to bring this on me." Another reported that: "Some of the more hurtful things that have been said to me have been from people in church where the attitude . . . at least some people have said to me, 'Well, all you have to do is just pick yourself up by the bootstraps. Just get off your duff and get going and it will take care of itself.' Or, 'You just don't have enough faith or you wouldn't feel like this. You just have to believe more. You have to pray more.'"

Thus, the discouraging message consumers experience is that they are both flawed and unworthy. Their symptoms do not trigger sympathy and support but elicit criticism and chastisement. As one consumer put it: "It's like you're a failure. You're a waste to human dignity or pride. And you're not worth anything. And you're worthless to society."

There were times, as well, when public reactions exceeded mere avoidance or failure to appreciate the reality of mental illness. At some times rejection was overt, deliberate, and even cruel. Several people who responded to our survey, for example, reported being deliberately harassed by others. "I have been called bad names by kids and teenagers in my community when they learned I had a mental illness," noted one consumer. "People called me things, like 'mentally retarded.' I've been called 'corn husker,' 'corn cob,' 'corn flakes,'. . . . I've been called a 'looney bird.'" Still another person experienced her neighbors' aggressive rejection: "Having lived eighteen years in one house, my neighbor found out about my illness. Called me crazy, threatened my family. Phone calls started, damage to property, and, after working with police, we needed to move. At the time I was working on my job of ten years on the Board of Directors of Head Start. The neighbors told their children to stay away from me— This is while I was teaching nursery school."

One person recounted the cruelty of his college classmates: "I was the subject of discrimination in college," wrote one man. "Because I had dark hair and brown eyes and was white and slender and built kind of lanky, I was given the name 'Norman,' as in 'Norman Bates' from the Hitchcock movie *Psycho*. At times half the dormitory population, twenty of the forty young men, would shout this name at me while emerging en masse from the building's elevator, and at nearly every other occasion."

Finally, another student described a heart-breaking incident:

> There was a young woman in several of my art classes . . . who would never miss a chance to insult me in some oblique way. . . . One day this individual [showed up] majorly stoned on marijuana. She sat down and started singing the words 'I'm a looney tune, I'm a looney tune" in a falsetto. I laughed along with everybody else at first, until I realized that some people looked embarrassed, some were smirking, and some were watching me very carefully and very quietly. I suddenly 'got it.' I realized the 'joke' was not about her state of 'stonedness' but rather the fact that apparently it had gotten around that I was an ex-mental patient. I had considered most of these people as 'friendly acquaintances,' and I was so shocked, I just sat there and pretended I didn't know that *I* was the joke.

As a mental health professional myself, I am embarrassed to report that consumers also experienced rejection at the hands of health- and mental health-care professionals. A common criticism of the mental health field has been that its theories sometimes blame consumers for their illnesses (and for not recovering speedily enough—as in popular term "treatment resistant" to designate patients whose painful symptoms have not been relieved by the treatments provided). Asked one consumer angrily: "Do you call stigma statements that blame the person or his family for the illness? What about statements that we got this way through cowardice, or that our illness is just a cover-up for ugly things inside of us or a result of our inability to love another human being? If this is stigma, then many of the things I learned from the mental health system as a child, teen, and young adult would have to be called examples of stigma."

Consumers also reported being treated with lack of respect by their caregivers, who made snide, patronizing, and offensive comments. One person described a consultation with a physician about chest pains that she feared might be a side effect of her medication; after confiding additional concerns that she was often getting angry, she reported, the doctor laughingly told her: "If you go on a shooting spree, be sure you don't come to *this office.*" Another consumer, who noted pointedly that "the worst discrimination I've faced *is from so-called mental health professionals,*" described one counselor who told her that her life was "a dirty, four letter word," while another counselor laughed at her when she recounted her previous suicidal impulses. Still another reported that his/her vocational rehabilitation counselor openly declared that "I would much rather work with a developmentally disabled client than a mentally ill client." In addition, many consumers who worked in mental health settings were aware that they were not entirely welcome in those roles, while others described instances in which their opinions and concerns were ignored or not taken seriously by health professionals (these dismissals are described in more detail in chapter 5).

I do not want to leave readers with the impression that everything was bleak for all consumers who communicated to us. Many positive experiences of support and understanding were described. Of our respondents, 83 percent were able to say that friends had been at least sometimes understanding or supportive; 47 percent said they had experienced this often or very often. In contrast to the tales of rejection many stories described support, particularly from friends and family, and made clear how valuable—and valued—such support can be: "I'd like to say that my parents are wonderful about my illness," wrote one survey respondent. "They've both been there from the beginning and during times I was manic they stuck by me despite what I did. . . . Thanks to wonderful new medicines and the fantastic support of my family I can face each day and live it as best I can." "Friends would come to see me in the hospital even though a mental hospital is not the funnest place in the world," said another. "They would come and see me. They would talk with me. . . . [Their support] means everything. They've actually saved my life in some circumstances." A third similarly detailed the importance of friendship for her:

> I have a friend that . . . just happened to be a Tupperware manager; that's how we met. And I ended up becoming a dealer for her for a while. But even when I stopped, it seemed like our contact never stopped even though she knew the trouble and

stuff that I was going through. She was right there. I could call her. I could talk with her. I could go to her house and visit. She has children, [but] she wasn't afraid to let me alone with her children. It was really good. It was nice. . . . She was just always there. . . . I'll never forget her for that 'cuz I really felt like I was alone in the world. I didn't feel like anybody cared. But when she came along, it gave me a little bit of hope of letting me know that at least one person cared about what happened to me. I'm very, very thankful for her.

When consumers found acceptance rather than rejection—sometimes much to their surprise and relief—it was a memorable and recovery-enhancing event for them. For example, one consumer described this: "I somehow dragged my 'defective self' through eight years of life after my first hospitalization before I took the risk to disclose to a new friend that I had had a mental illness. I remember bracing myself for his obvious reaction—surprise, loathing, and rejection. When his response came, my empowerment process began. He said something like, 'Oh, do you still want to get together for lunch tomorrow?' To feel that I was being viewed as a human and not just a disease, to see that my incredibly high fears were fantasized paranoia about the consequences of disclosure, that real moment was worth more than any amount of therapy."

Finally, to appreciate fully how much simple acceptance can mean to consumers I include this account of another woman's unexpected success: "I've lived in Board-and-Care homes, and it's just not for me. They're real awful. . . . [So] I answered an ad when I was in the hospital in the local newspaper for room and board in exchange for light services. And I was interviewed for that when I got discharged from the hospital, and they liked me, and I moved in with this lovely family in this very nice area. I didn't tell them I was mentally ill. They had an old lady mother who was just darling, and they just wanted someone in and out and that was fine because I was going to day care. I didn't tell them. I just told them I was playing tennis and stuff that I would be in and out." Unfortunately, the woman, a sufferer from depression, eventually became despondent and called a suicide prevention agency which, in turn, sent the police to the house.

Knowing that the police intervention would force her to reveal her mental illness, the woman "went upstairs and packed up my suitcase to leave. And this couple came in, and I was crying and they said 'What happened?'. . . . So then I had to tell [them] that I was mentally ill and that I would leave in the morning. So they went into the library and they came back and they said 'We'd like you to stay here.' And I was there for three years, and it was wonderful. I got very well. I got my real estate license and a job selling real estate. . . . It was just a wonderful experience. I'm blessed to have had that."

It is certainly encouraging and important to recognize that such positive experiences can and do occur. One might also take comfort from the fact that more than one-third (38 percent) of consumers responding to our survey reported that they have seldom or never been shunned or avoided by others when their consumer status was revealed, and nearly half (46 percent) saw themselves as having often or very often been treated fairly by others who knew of their mental illnesses. These same figures, however, also mean that the *majority* of consumers did *not* find fair treatment a common occurrence and *had* experienced shunning and rejection with some frequency. In fact, even within some grateful descriptions of social support and acceptance consumers had received, there was the implicit message that this sort of experience, important and satisfying as it was, did not happen nearly often enough. "I have one coworker in particular who is very accepting of my depression," noted one consumer. "I use the word accept in the best possible way. She harbors no pity, few preconceived notions, and absolutely no hostility for me based on this condition. I only wish that I felt there were more people like her."

Overall, then, consumer feedback confirms what would be predicted from public attitude research: mental illness brings social rejection and isolation to many who suffer from it. The stories of consumers also help us to appreciate the many, sometimes subtle or unintended, ways rejection is communicated and the many sources through which it comes. The observations of consumers reveal that they are well aware of the discomfort and fear that others experience around them and therefore seek to avoid. Old friends are lost, and new ones become difficult to acquire when it is known that the person has a mental illness. Even families and clergy sometimes fail to provide needed support; they reveal a lack of acceptance of mental illness as a "real" disorder, which leads to victim blaming and attributing problems to character or moral failure, which only further increases consumers' sense of rejection. Harassment, insult, and cruel teasing are also part of consumers' experience, sometimes from mental health caregivers themselves. It is small wonder, then, that one consumer observed: "it is people shunning me that makes me feel so low and unworthy."

5

Discouragement

and Lowered

Goals

To help educate students from my classes about mental illness, I often encourage them to volunteer at psychiatric treatment facilities over an extended period of time to get to know the people receiving services there. Student reactions have confirmed my belief that this is a valuable learning experience. One student, for example, returned from his weekly visit to a psychiatric hospital with this account: He had gone to the facility's recreation room with a resident he had been visiting regularly, and the two played several games of table tennis, a game at which the student considered himself quite skilled. To the student's amazement, this patient beat him handily. The student was learning what many fail to understand—a person who has mental illness is not necessarily impaired in all areas of functioning.

The student's surprise that his opponent, despite his severe mental illness, could show such a high level of proficiency in table tennis reflects a common experience for mental health consumers: their overall competence is doubted, as if all skills, knowledge, and sensibilities are removed by mental illness. Of the respondents to our survey, 70 percent, in fact, indicated that they had at least sometimes been treated as less competent when others learned of their mental illness. To more than one-third (36 percent), this had happened often or very often.

It is appropriate to acknowledge, of course, that the treatment of people with mental illness as having diminished competence is not entirely without some basis in reality. Sometimes mental illnesses do disrupt behavior and interfere significantly with consumers' ability to perform specific tasks. Mental illnesses, particularly severe mental illnesses *may* interfere with intellectual functioning, as well. They may impair the person's judgment and distort his/her perceptions. They may make concentration, reasoning, and decision making more difficult. They may contribute to impaired performance on intelligence tests and academic examinations. Medications that consumers take, moreover, may impair their speech and slow their thoughts and movement. All these things provide some basis for people observing consumers to conclude that their abilities are limited.

To anticipate a high level of inability *primarily* on the basis of a psychiatric label or based solely on the knowledge that the person has had psychiatric treatment, however, is inappropriate. Many consumers, even with severe mental illness, are extraordinarily competent and accomplished. Nobel Prize–winner John Nash, actress Patty Duke, Pulitzer Prize–winning author William Styron, and the late Florida Senator and Governor Lawton Chiles are just a few of the well-known people with mental illnesses whose talent and success challenge the presumption of incompetence.[1] Thousands, if not millions, of others demonstrate everyday competencies, like the rest of the population, in managing their lives, meeting job requirements, and finding productive outlets for their energy. What consumers were most concerned about, then, was the almost automatic, stereotypical *assumption* of lacking competence. They were distressed that others seemed simply to assume, because of the consumer's label or treatment history, that he or she was fragile and incapable. They were concerned that, instead of recognizing the possibility of substantial variation—between individuals and across time—in degree of impairment and basing their assessments on the performance and needs of the individual consumer at the current point in their recovery, people reacted as if all with a mental health label have a uniformly high degree of inability.

One common complaint, for example, was that people behaved

as if mental illness were the same as mental retardation. Mental retardation, of course, refers to lifelong limitations of intellect that in turn translate into limitations on learning; mental illness, however, typically refers to a spectrum of psychiatric conditions that interfere with an individual's usual or prior level of functioning.[2] People of all intellectual abilities are vulnerable to mental illness; thus, some people with mental illness also have mental retardation. Similarly, some people with mental retardation also have mental illnesses. But the two are as independent as visual and hearing impairments; one may have both, but there is no reason to assume that a person who has one also has the other.

Nevertheless, many consumers found themselves treated as if their having a mental illness also meant they were very limited in intelligence. "Many still believe," observed one consumer, "that neurobiological disorders are the same as mental retardation. Although I had a 4.0 average in law school, I now often find others explaining concepts to me as if I were a five-year-old." Another stated, "People talk more slowly to me as if I'm stupid." Still another noted angrily that "although I was a National Merit Scholar, I was told I am 'not college material' and, on three occasions, declared 'retarded.'" One woman discerned the low expectations of her abilities from the surprise she encountered when she succeeded at a challenging task: "It seems like people assume that I'm stupid because I have a mental health problem. . . . I run a web page for an organization which is a consumer-run support organization for people with dissociative disorders. And like the Center for Mental Health is astounded that a consumer could create this web page. Well, that's my job. I work in information technology, and I'm very good at what I do, and just because I have a dissociative disorder doesn't mean that I'm stupid."

Although the consumers in our survey tended to be both well-educated and highly accomplished (almost one in five had completed college and gone on to graduate or professional degrees), many found themselves talked down to, patronized, and treated like children by others. "Some people talk down to you," said one interviewee, "make things real simple. I feel like pulling out my college degree. It just seems like sometimes people think that you can't be intelligent. I'm supposed to be stupid I guess." Another described being spoken to in a disrespectful manner, "babied . . . pitied, condescending tones, treated as if I had no intellect." Numerous others noted similar condescending treatment: "Typically, I am treated as though I am invisible. On other occasions, I am treated as if I had limited intelligence. I am talked down to quite often." "It's just like instead of talking to an adult they're talking to a child. . . . I have a lot of trouble at doctors' offices. The minute they see the bipolar disorder diagnosis, they immediately, instantly think that you're not with it and talk down to you." "People leave me no room to prove my own competencies and have treated me with less mental ability in my actions and qualifications and therefore don't give me a chance to prove my own abilities or competencies. In this process, they assume things that are not true and talk down to me, especially when it comes to my qualifications."

The assumption of limited ability was so strong that even the known abilities of consumers were disregarded. "In high school, my IQ was rated at 136," observed one person. "People who used to view me as intelligent now question even general statements that I make." Those who were respected and valued reported that they lost that respect after mental illness. One woman reported:

> I'm the mother of five. I took good care of my kids for years. No complaints, no nothing. I was president of an adoptive parents group. People came to me for advice. I was ombudsman on my husband's ship; when women had problems they came to me for help. . . . When I got out [of the hospital after treatment for depression] . . . someone from church happened to call me and began giving parenting advice. And it wasn't supportive parenting advice. It was very basic bonehead parenting stuff, you know, that you might say to a fifteen-year-old. It was extremely patronizing. And it's like suddenly I'm incompetent because I was in the hospital.

Such patronizing and condescension came from not only those with little knowledge of mental illness, but also mental health professionals. Similar to the experiences of Rosenhan's pseudopatients, described in chapter 2, mental health staff were reported as talking down to patients as if they were unintelligent children. "Mental health professionals don't seem to know how to treat me or communicate with me without being condescending," wrote one consumer, "or not take me seriously, talk down to me." "Some of the staff members [at a group home]," reported another, "treat the residents as if they are children, talk down to them, etc., thus lowering the residents' self-esteem." A third complained that mental health caregivers "figure if you're mentally ill, you have a second-grade education, you're illiterate, you're stupid. . . . They don't figure you can be something and still be mentally ill."

When mental health treatment history was revealed, consumers found that inabilities of all kinds were assumed. Much like my student who initially expected that mental illness impaired even things like table tennis skill, people seemed to assume a wide range of inabilities when mental health treatment history was revealed. Consumers' ability to make responsible financial judgments was doubted, for instance. "When I went to the Social Security office upon approval of my claim, I was told to bring an adult family member with me," wrote a well-educated adult respondent from our survey. "Upon our arrival, my husband was told that he would be my 'representative payee,' but nothing in my records said that I had any difficulty handling our finances." Another person, who had been church trustee, steward, and superintendent of a Sunday school, described how his demonstrated leadership and business abilities were suddenly called into question by a psychiatric disorder: "When the people in my congregation in church found out that I had a psychiatric disorder . . . our pastor and the chairman of the trustee and steward board came to me and asked, 'Since you had your crisis, do you think that you are still qualified to render business decisions?'" Even the ability to relate in a loving way to grandchildren was placed in doubt by mental illness, according to one woman: "My son and daughter-in-law will not allow me to keep my three-year-old granddaughter (but my niece lets me sit for her two-year- and five-month-old children and I do fine). I have never been negligent. I am allowed to see my granddaughter once every five to six weeks with my son present only."

Messages about assumed lack of competence came also from having job and other responsibilities taken away or reduced following one's illness. Over and over, people described how revelation of psychiatric disorder led to diminished responsibilities: "I think that once people find out that I'm a consumer, they ask less of me or expect less of me. When nobody knows that I have this diagnosis, then I seem to get the same share of responsibilities as anyone else." "I have had coworkers think I'm less capable of doing some office work and often end up with the more menial jobs," reported another. Even the ability to participate in a task as minimally arduous (and potentially therapeutic) as baking cookies was questioned, according to still another consumer: "At church," she reported, "I have not been asked to do jobs when people knew I was in depression again. . . . That cookie baking or committee assignment would have been therapy for me, but they thought depression is caused by overwork."

Again, one could argue that the responses of people in the above examples are well-founded in the known vulnerabilities of people with mental illnesses—and well-intended as way to protect vulnerable individuals from unhealthy burdens. Mental illnesses *are* exacerbated by stress, and they may make the individual more fragile, in the sense of their being more vulnerable to stress. Sometimes, in fact, consumers themselves often call for patience and understanding of the limitations imposed by their disorders. However, consumers, like most nonconsumers, also want opportunities and challenges, and, to those consumers, the automatic assumption of decreased competence was experienced as condescending and dispiriting. "A few people have acted as though I don't have a brain," summarized one of our respondents. "This is demeaning."

Moreover, assumptions of fragility and decreased competence, however protectively intended, sometimes even increased stress, as consumers felt not only devalued but under uncomfortable scrutiny. When their mental illness or treatment was known, consumers sometimes were aware that others were watching them carefully to be sure that the job would not be too much for them and that they were not breaking down under the pressure. "There's always sort of this change in attitude [when consumer status is revealed]," observed one interviewee, "like maybe you can't really do that job, maybe you weren't really cut out for it. I struggled for a long time to try to become chairman of the human rights committee at the local hospital. And finally when it came about . . . I always felt that I had to prove who I was and what I was doing and that I could really cope with the responsibility." Another noted: "I was in a nursing position in a doctor's office, and I told them in the beginning that I had depression, and they questioned a lot of things I did. They would watch me. . . . They questioned me about certain things, and if I didn't know the answers, they just kinda looked disgusted then. [I felt] humiliated, discouraged, and down on myself." Two consumers we heard from even had to formally prove themselves through psychiatric examination: "I am a professional [an attorney] and have been required by my partners to undergo an independent psychiatric examination concerning my ability to continue in my career and to do my job once I told them about my [bipolar] diagnosis." "I go through hell and back each year with my annual physical, having to obtain letters from my psychiatrist, primary care doctor and therapist that I'm capable of doing a job I've been doing for eight years! Also I had to obtain letters from three psychiatrists when I applied to go to school to become a psychiatric technician. It was assumed I couldn't handle the stress."

Consumers also found burdensome the tendency of others to interpret their behavior in terms of their disorders, implicitly communicating an expectancy of incompetence. Because consumers are assumed incompetent, almost any lapse, they find, is attributed to their illnesses. Brief memory lapses, temporary confusion, or uncertainty—such as everyone experiences from time to time—take on different interpretations when the person has a history of mental illness. A pause, for example, may be seen as evidence that one is having trouble finishing a thought. As one consumer noted: "Often, while serving on panels as speaker, I find myself interrupted in mid-sentence by a family member or provider in an attempt to finish a sentence for me. Very frustrating." Another complained that: "My illness is always pulled out in front of me. If I can't remember something for a split second, I hear 'the mind is always the first thing to go.' You get the picture here. The diagnosed mentally ill person is not allowed to have the same lapses in memory or behavior that others [can]. He is *forever* stigmatized, labeled, and branded." One woman lamented that consumers cannot even be given credit for their own human errors: "I had a house fire several years ago, which unfortunately was my fault, but it was carelessness, not a product of my illness. But that was not the implication that was made. The implication was made that it had something to do with my being mentally ill." Another woman reported similarly that an uncharacteristic deviation from her otherwise fastidious personal appearance— her slip was showing—had the result that people "looked at me like that's part of the illness. They read into things that just aren't there." While, on the one hand, such attitudes may be seen as giving the consumer more leeway—lapses are more easily forgiven when one simply attributes them to the illness—on the other hand, the implicit message is that such lapses are to be expected from a mental patient; they simply reflect that consumer's unavoidable incompetence.

Even the sympathetic concerns of friends and families were sometimes experienced by consumers as a demonstration of typical lack of faith in their abilities. "I feel my brother and mother, to some degree, think I'm fragile in some way," explained one consumer, "even though I've worked every day of my life and have supported my wife of the past six years." "I've found many people start to treat me as if I were made of glass after finding out about my condition," wrote another. "They feel they need to shield me and are hyperconcerned about my every change of mood." Still another group observed: "Others treat me differently, as if I am going to fall apart if they say the 'wrong thing' to me." "I have sometimes been treated like I might fall apart if exposed to any stress whatsoever."

Once more it is important to recognize that much of this objectionable behavior of friends, family, and coworkers described is probably well-intended. People sincerely believe they are helping by speaking more calmly and slowly to consumers, reducing their workload, and relieving them from responsibilities. Nevertheless, from the viewpoint of consumers—and that is the viewpoint with which our study and this book is primarily concerned—the reactions to them as mental health consumers were belittling and discouraging; they communicated lack of confidence in them as capable human beings. As one consumer expressed it: "Even the people that try to help us . . . treat us as though we're helpless and they try to protect us too much. Because they believe that we're unable to help ourselves. That message is not a healthy one."

In many instances in which consumers described messages of incompetence, however, even benign intent was hard to find. Occasionally, for instance, such messages were both explicit and harsh. "In August 1995, within one week of returning from a leave of absence for treatment of depression, I was called into the director's office," reported one concerned worker. "At that time, I was encouraged to voluntarily resign my nursing position, which I had held for nine years. She said 'mental illness makes people squeamish.' She also then said that she 'could guarantee me that I wasn't going to be able to cut the mustard.'"

Consumers also found themselves being disregarded, ignored, and treated as if their ideas (coming, as they do, from a person with mental illness) were of little value. Because consumers are viewed incapable of contributing in useful ways, they have long been excluded from treatment and mental health system planning. That view is slowly changing, but consumer experiences suggest they still find it difficult to be heard and taken seriously. "When you are a consumer," lamented one survey participant, "NO ONE in the mental health community *listens* to you. You are immediately deemed incompetent and stupid." This experience was echoed by other consumers as well: "[You are] stigmatized even in the county system. No validity. Lack of respect. They listen with one ear, and they don't think you have anything of value to say." "Because I believed I was communicating with my brother who is dead . . . they assumed that I had nothing to say and that all my thoughts were deranged, which was not true at all. I had plenty to say, and there were plenty of my thoughts that were not deranged. . . . It's just assumed . . . that nothing I had to say on any level was of any significance at any time. That I couldn't speak coherently, intelligently on my behalf or anybody else's." "People who know I am different from them in some way either talk down to me in simple language or talk to others as if I were not in the room. They make decisions for me or about what I can do or not do without even asking me what I think about what I should do."

The legitimate opinions and emotions of consumers were sometimes discredited in other contexts as well. It was apparent that consumers who become upset and express their anger, sadness, confusion, and so on, are often seen as merely displaying the symptoms of their disorders; the possibility that they may have good reason to be upset is not considered—and thus the source of that upset is often not addressed. One consumer, for instance, noted that her reactions are often discredited with the question, "Have you taken your medication?" "Others may be just as silly, crazy, and they don't hear that statement," the respondent astutely observed.

Consumers' opinions (especially if they are contrary to what others think) may be discounted as the product of a disordered, illogical, or emotionally unstable mind. "When I disagree with remarks [made by my family]," noted one consumer, "they almost always remind me of my illness." "I have a master's degree in social work," said another, "and one would think that would assure my competence. Wrong. I work for a state mental health authority . . . and my competence is routinely questioned. . . . If I'm not exactly with the party line, it's because I'm a consumer. . . . And the term is always '*just* a consumer.' If I ask too many questions . . . it's 'Are you feeling well today? Have you talked with your psychiatrist?' Very demeaning." Still another survey respondent said: "If what I decide to do for myself doesn't agree with what these people think I ought to be doing, then their only conclusion is that it must be coming from some part of me that's still really sick. . . . I'm not given room for my own ideas. I'm not given credit for some parts of me that might actually be together." As articulated by Esso Leete in a 1994 issue of the *Journal of the California Alliance for the Mentally Ill*, such experiences leave consumers feeling disregarded: "I can talk, but I may not be heard. I can make suggestions, but they may not be taken seriously. I can report my thoughts, but they may be seen as delusions. I can recite experiences, but they may be interpreted as fantasies. To be a patient is to be discounted."[3]

Another area of significant consequence for consumers was their dismissal by physicians: once their psychiatric diagnosis or medication history was known, their medical complaints were not taken seriously. Anecdotal reports of physicians who do not pay proper attention to their patients' complaints are frustratingly frequent in today's society, and those with psychiatric disorders are among the most vulnerable to being disregarded. A psychiatric history may lead easily to the assumption that somatic complaints are imagined or are part of the mental illness and thus not to be considered seriously. One consumer, for instance, reported:

> I went to the doctor from my HMO plan. I was just feeling real confused . . . but it did not feel like my normal symptoms at all. And I had bronchitis at the time and I was taking some kind of cough syrup to help me sleep, and it had either codeine or some kind of different form of codeine synthetic, and I really felt like this was making me feel very strange. So I did go to the doctor to find out what was going on. And he knew my history and immediately discounted me. And was like, "Well, you have a mental illness, so that explains all of it." And I kept trying to tell him that this was not one of my regular symptoms because I know what they are by now and this is different and I think it is this medication. And he was just not willing to listen to that at all. So I went home and discontinued it, and the next day I was fine.

This lack of credibility with physicians not only discouraged consumers, but sometimes it produced serious physical consequences. One respondent described how she had "walked on a fractured foot for two months and went to three doctors before a doctor took me seriously, x-rayed my foot, and put a cast on it. I couldn't believe what I read in my charts about fictitious pain due to depression." Another explained: "When you have to tell [doctors] what medication you are taking . . . they treat you differently and a lot of physical complaints are written off as being 'just in your head' or that you create your physical illness. And so after a while you learn to just live with pain and the things that are wrong with you because you know that if you go to the doctors they are just going to write you off anyway. . . . I had a severe cramp and that was written off as being psychosomatic when in fact I had a severe case of endometriosis and had to have a hysterectomy. But for many years no one paid attention to my pain."

Similar experiences occurred in the context of psychiatric treatment. One person, for instance, described this experience while in a psychiatric hospital: "I kept telling this doctor that came through once a week that something was wrong. My hands were all swollen to the point where I couldn't wear gloves. And he said, 'Well, it's not the Mellaril; that's not a side effect" And then one day I stood up and I passed out and my blood pressure was 80 over 50. So they took me off the Mellaril and three days later I was fine. They just don't believe you; they just discount." A similar story came from a research analyst who was being treated for depression: "[My psychiatrist] had me on Nardil, which was causing me all kinds of falling episodes. And I kept telling her I was falling at my home all the time and hitting my head on things, and she would just keep increasing the dosage. . . . And the final fall was when I was trying to get to my telephone quickly in my kitchen fairly early in the morning and slipped and fell twice on my ankle in the same spot and sustained a severe compound fracture. . . . It's just incredible that it took a compound fracture and surgery to be listened to."

Psychiatric status fuels this kind of neglect from physicians; the neglect is glaring in instances when the consumer achieved proper attention only when a nonconsumer became involved. "I stated I felt two lumps, which doctors ignored," reported one woman. "Six months later, at my sister's insistence, a doctor did a biopsy. . . . Three kinds of cancer were found." The delayed diagnosis and advanced condition required the woman to have a mastectomy, and she now says: "I feel stigma and discrimination *have* compromised and will continue to compromise the quality of my medical care." Consumers also reported that the quality of their treatment varied depending on whether or not they identified themselves (or were identified by their treatment/medication history) as consumers. One consumer wrote: "I went in [to an emergency room] being honest re all the meds I was on. Terrible treatment. Went in eight months later. Didn't reveal meds. Made up story about being from out of town. . . . I was treated as gold by many I'd seen eight months ago. In order to receive good medical care one must be dishonest to the medical profession. VERY SAD! ANGER ESCALATES. DEPRESSION DEEPENS." The irony is not to be missed here: Physicians doubt the honesty and accuracy of consumers' symptom reports; thus, the only way to have symptoms accepted as honest and accurate reports is to be dishonest about psychiatric history.

Not only is medical care compromised by physician skepticism about the medical complaints of people with psychiatric histories, but patients are insulted and belittled by such attitudes. An incident recounted at the 1997 Rosalynn Carter Symposium on Mental Health Policy, although not from a consumer in our survey, is worthy of retelling for its demonstration of how physician attitudes can change from helpful interest in the patient's reported problem to infuriating questioning of those same symptoms once information about psychiatric treatment is discovered or disclosed: The young woman described how she had chipped a tooth and taken some Tylenol-with-codeine to relieve the pain until she could get to a dentist. Unfortunately, she began to have a possibly allergic reaction to the medicine. Her heart began to pound with sufficient intensity that she went quickly to an emergency room. She explained to the attending physician that she had taken the Tylenol and feared she was having a bad reaction to it. When asked if she had ever experienced heart symptoms before, she answered honestly in the affirmative and noted that her treatment had been at the same hospital. The physician then accessed her medical record to check on this previous treatment. It became obvious when he returned, however, that he had also discovered in her record that she had had prior psychiatric treatment, as well. It was obvious because, this woman noted, the nature and manner of his questioning changed.

Now he asked very deliberately,

"What did you take?"
"Tylenol with codeine," she told him again.
"And how many pills did you take?"
"One."
"Are you sure it was just one?"
"Yes, just one."
"And why did you take this medicine?"
"Because I chipped a tooth," she explained with increasing exasperation, "and I'm not really fond of mouth pain."

And while that explanation might have been sufficient had the woman not had a history of psychiatric treatment, the physician added yet another indignity. "Show me the tooth," he said, communicating clearly that her word was not good enough to be accepted without proof.

Assumptions about consumers' incompetence and inability to handle stress also led to another problem for consumers—advice to lower expectations in life. More than half (56 percent) of the consumer respondents to our survey reported that they had at least sometimes been advised to lower their expectations in life because of their mental illness; for more than one in four (27 percent), this had occurred often or very often. "My mama said I have a high expectation," said one consumer. "She told me to lower it because it's getting too high, and it's going to get out of hand. And my cousin told me the same thing. When I was at Shoneys, I would do stuff, like I'm going to have another job, I'm going to be a supervisor. And then she said, you better lower your expectations because that might never happen. . . . I felt real bad about it because I thought I always could do more than I was doing at Shoneys." Another woman described her understanding of the messages she was receiving: "The implication is there. There's no point in going through with [school plans] because (a) you won't finish it, (b) you'll get tired, bored, whatever, and your grades will come down. . . . Where it comes to employment, 'Well, you're not going to be able to put up with their rules and regulations, so why bother?' In other words, go take some stupid minimum wage job flipping burgers."

Frequently advice to lower expectations took the form of exhortations to "be realistic," and the advice often came from mental health caregivers. "I was in a day program for nearly two years that kept telling me 'to face reality,'" reported a typical respondent. "I had a mental illness and would never be able to work or participate in normal life again." "It is ironic," observed another similarly, "that psychiatrists often overplay problems and urge you to expect less of yourself. The language is 'you must realize your limitations'—real or imaginary. Then when you accomplish what they did not expect of you, they are amazed."

Consumers were further troubled by the treatment programs they encountered that set limited goals for them and actively discouraged them from pursuing higher goals. Said one person: "One [vocational rehabilitation program] counselor told me, because I was in a state hospital, why should I have any competence and no, they wouldn't send me to school. Their programs were to train you to be a janitor. . . . They treat consumers like mentally retarded a lot, assuming that they don't have intelligence or the capabilities to do much more." Another described a similar experience: "I've gone to state rehab services. I told them I'd like to take courses in being a computer operator of some sort, like databases and stuff like that and they said the only thing I'm good for is clearing out toilets." A third lamented that "My case manager will say, 'Well, you better not take too much of a load or go to school because you might be causing too much stress.' . . . I've had case managers hint not to push for the highest accomplishments I can do. . . . Sometimes it would be nice if they would push for something more than just sitting in chairs all day." Still another reported, "I have been told by members of a support group that I should stock shelves instead of continuing with my search for a position in the profession for which I trained." One woman with bipolar disorder was even discouraged from considering parenthood: "I've had people tell me not to have children because it will probably be too much stress on my body and because of my illness."

Once again, it is possible to see these messages as well-intended and sometimes even helpful. Recovery can, in fact, be set back if consumers hurry to undertake stressful and demanding tasks that then overwhelm them. Just as it would not be wise for persons recovering from heart attacks to immediately begin or renew strenuous exercise, recovering consumers may need to maintain a gradual pace for their recovery. Just as medical patients, wishing to deny their limitations, often make poor judgments about what postillness activities to undertake, psychiatric patients may show similar inclinations, sometimes exacerbated by thinking and planning impairments imposed by their illnesses. Cautions about setting realistic goals may be necessary and helpful to consumers inclined to push too fast in their recovery.

The concern of consumers, however, is that the goals that others see for them as "realistic" are often *unrealistically* low, based upon others' inaccurate stereotypes of incompetence and fragility. Even the severe mental illnesses of schizophrenia and bipolar disorder no longer warrant the poor prognoses they had twenty-five years ago.

Improved medications and innovative social and community programs have enabled individuals with these disorders to recover and resume productive roles in their communities. Many of these individuals, in fact, have been instrumental in developing and running some of the most successful psychiatric rehabilitation programs. The expectations of others, however, including many mental health caregivers, seem to have lagged behind these advances, such that caregivers tend to greatly underestimate the potential of consumers, as shown by the story of one respondent who proudly recounted how she had overcome the limited expectations of her therapist: "I was seeing this one psychiatrist, and he told me I would never work. He told me just to accept that I'm going to have to be at home and in and out of hospitals. [He] told me that I was chronically mentally ill. That I had an IQ of 79 and just to go home and live with it. . . . I was angry. And I was determined to show him that I could work. Since he told me that, I went back to graduate school, got an MSW, and [now] I'm working three days a week at a mental health substance abuse clinic."

This last consumer's career choice touches an area of particular controversy with respect to consumer competence and discouragement from pursuing goals—work in the mental health field. Many consumers, because of their own experiences with mental illness, had strong desires to become involved with mental health work. They felt that they had enhanced understanding of mental health issues as a result of their own struggles with mental illness, wanted to help others with similar problems, and/or wanted to return something to the mental health field out of gratitude for the help they had received. Consumers, then, often sought opportunities to work as mental health caregivers themselves. What they commonly encountered were skepticism about their abilities to handle such work, opinions that their "mental instability" automatically disqualified them for work with psychiatric populations, and policies that prohibited their hiring (or even their acceptance as volunteers). "One teacher at my school," reported a consumer who had returned to college after being treated for a psychiatric disorder, "believes that I am unable to fulfill my future duties as a psychologist just because he knows I have a psychiatric diagnosis. (So far as I know, he is unaware of what it is.) I have a 3.6 average." Another reported: "Ironically, some of the worst treatment I have received has been at the hands of the graduate school of social work I am currently enrolled in. For instance, one of my professors was told (referring to me) by a school administrator that 'we (the department) don't know if mentally ill students should be allowed to work with other mentally ill people.' Ironic, since that's what I do for a living."

Certainly, the mental health field cannot be faulted for its caution about whom it employs to work with people in crisis. Assisting people with mental illnesses requires great skill and confers a high degree of responsibility. It has long been a tenet of psychiatry that those who are too absorbed in or impaired by their own psychological dilemmas will not be able to maintain the attention and objectivity necessary to meet the needs of others in mental distress. However, once again, the stereotype-based generalizations apparent in judgments about fitness for psychiatric work are objectionable. Many successful clinicians have suffered from mental illnesses, among them Kay Jamison, a leading clinician and researcher in the area of bipolar disorder and herself a longtime sufferer of that illness, and Fred Frese, a psychologist who rose to the rank of director of a large psychiatric hospital despite periodic episodes of schizophrenic symptoms.[4] As noted previously, many of the most successful community programs have been created and overseen by consumers. Many respondents to our survey are now working in the mental health field. Obviously, the assumption that consumers are too unstable or incompetent to work in mental health is untrue.

Not only did messages to lower expectations underestimate consumer potential, but they were sometimes delivered in harsh and dramatically discouraging words. One interviewee, for example, described how the first doctor who diagnosed her bipolar disorder instructed her that "people with your problem will have a very low level type of life." Another explained how his aspirations were thrown back in his face as evidence of his disorder: "I have been told I was delusional in hoping to better myself while under skilled psychiatric nursing care in my home by the Registered Nurse treating me. He told me that my speech patterns revealed a thought disorder that would mean I should prudently enter a life care community rather than hope for a meaningful education." Still another reported: "Once a psychiatrist said he didn't know anything I'd be good for, until I showed him some examples [of my artwork]. Then he allowed that 'Well, maybe you'd be worth saving after all.'" Perhaps this last psychiatrist was trying to be humorous, but his remarks left a lasting—and unfavorable—impression.

Overall, then, consumer comments reveal that people with mental illnesses experience frequent devaluation and discouragement. Others treat them as if their disorders render them unintelligent and incapable of living, working, and achieving at the same level of others. They find their opinions, their emotions, even their medical complaints discounted and ignored. They are treated as excessively fragile, helpless, and incapable of handling stresses; they are accordingly overprotected and relieved of job and other responsibilities even when they have demonstrated competence in fulfilling such duties. They are advised—often by knowledgeable mental health experts and often in a rather blunt and insensitive manner—that they are less able than others and that they need to accept lives far below their aspirations. Such experiences leave consumers longing for hope and respect, like this one who wrote: "I want so much to have the veil of stigma lifted, to be taken seriously again, like I was as a respected lecturer and presenter before small groups or thousands in conventions. I want to be thought of as one who may have radical ideas and revolutionary ways of doing things, without manic depression perceived as the reason or cause."

6

Discrimination

When someone is denied an opportunity for which he or she is qualified based on membership in a particular religious, ethnic, racial, or gender group, that is discrimination. Decisions to hire someone, for example, must, by law, be based on the prospective employee's ability to do the job, not on his or her age, gender, race, and so forth. Sometimes, however, discrimination is difficult for employers to recognize because prejudices and stereotypes may influence their assessment of an applicant's ability to do the job. An employer who believes that women are hormonally and emotionally unsuited to hard-nosed corporate work may wrongly believe that the female applicant is indeed less able to do the job than a male applicant and thus believes that the decision not to hire her is based, as required, on job-related criteria. Such a decision, based on false stereotypes, is nevertheless discrimination. An employer who does not hire African-Americans because he falsely believes that blacks are lazy and unreliable—and thus wrongly views them as poor workers—is discriminating.

The 1990 Americans with Disabilities Act (ADA) makes it clear that exclusion of qualified individuals based on disability—including mental disability—is also discrimination and therefore illegal.[1] An employer who makes employment decisions about someone in a wheelchair or someone with a visual impairment without regard to the person's ability to fulfill the specific job requirements is discriminating. If an employer denies a job to someone based on his stereotypes of disabled workers rather than on their demonstrated qualifications, that is discrimination. Similarly, if an employer turns down otherwise qualified job applicants because they have had prior psychiatric treatment (based on his inaccurate belief that a person with a mental health problem cannot be a good employee), that is discrimination. Such discrimination was encountered by many of the mental health consumers responding to our survey.

Approximately one in three respondents (31 percent) indicated that they had been turned down for a job for which they were qualified when their consumer status was revealed; half of these individuals (15 percent) said that this had occurred often or very often.[2] These results are similar to those of a 1965 study by Dorothy Miller and William Dawson. Interviewing 156 consumers returning to a psychiatric hospital following "a leave of absence," they reported that approximately half of their interviewees indicated that they believed their status as former hospital patients had created hardships for them in the community; a third of these expressed the view that their former patient status had directly prevented them from seeking, obtaining, or holding a job.[3] Difficulty obtaining a job was reported also in consumer studies by Don Spiegel and Jenny Younger in 1972 and by Link and his colleagues in 1997.[4] Employment discrimination against those with mental illnesses seems to be a long-standing tradition.

Whether being turned down for a job is discrimination, of course, can sometimes be difficult to determine. Mental illness often disrupts educational and vocational progress, and episodes of severe illness and perhaps accompanying hospitalizations leave gaps in work history about which prospective employers could legitimately be concerned. It is appropriate for employers to try to ascertain how reliable a worker will be, and work history is an appropriate criterion for this determination. As many of our respondents indicated, it is possible that they were turned down for some jobs because of not only their consumer status but also their poor employment histories. In addition, legitimate employment decisions are often made on the basis of interview impressions. Consumers applying for jobs who may have residual symptoms or whose interrupted development may have delayed the acquisition of needed impression management skills may not come across as the poised, confident candidate employers are seeking. A negative employment decision under such circumstances may not be discriminatory.

Thus, some job rejections reported by consumers may not have been job discrimination. However, it would be a mistake to assume that respondents in general were not differentiating between lack of success in getting a job and actual discrimination. As noted in the description of our survey instrument in chapter 3, we stressed on the questionnaire the distinction between being turned down for a job and being turned down *"on grounds unrelated to your competencies."* Furthermore, many consumers in our survey commented themselves on the difficulty of being sure if discrimination was the reason for their being turned down and seemed to be applying the discrimination label with caution. "It's hard to say DEFINITELY I've been turned down for jobs because of my illness," said one person, "but in no instance where I've levelled with my prospective employer about my condition have I gotten the job." "I could be wrong," said another, "but I don't think so."

Although consumers could not be positive that their illness was the deciding factor in their lack of success obtaining employment, it was hard to think otherwise when disclosure of their illness was so reliably followed by rejection as job applicants. "In job interviews, once they find out I'm on medications," reported one interviewee, "I'm usually dismissed. They don't give the reasons. But that's the reason." "When I'd look for work," reported another, "and people would ask if I had any problems and when (I didn't know any better at the time; I'd never dealt with this) I put down that I was manic-depressive. . . . They says 'Well, we've already got other candidates we're looking at for the job.' Even though I was qualified or more qualified for the job, and I'd be dismissed." Still another recalled: "I wanted to work part-time, and I went to this little [office]. They had ads in the paper. I applied. Was interviewed. . . . I did divulge to the girl that interviewed me that I had been in a psychiatric unit, that I was well on my way to recovery, that I could furnish her with a statement from my psychiatrist. . . . She said she would get in touch with me. I waited a few days. And three or four days later I went back to see the woman that had interviewed me and asked her why . . . she did not give me any consideration. I'd had everything available. Had even had training. She couldn't give me an answer. I knew the answer." One woman's prospective employer left even less room for inference about the cause of job denial: "I'm a licensed practical nurse. I went to a nursing home to see if I could get a full-time job with them, and my nursing qualifications were fine. But for myself I feel that it's important to let my employers know that yes I do have this problem but I am under treatment. As soon as this particular person found out that I had the mental health issue, she very politely told me that she felt it would be better that I find some other type of work to go to, that this would not be a very good environment for me to be in. And basically, showed me to the door."

The change of attitude of interviewers and prospective employers when psychiatric status was disclosed, as well as the negative outcomes, helped to convince consumers that their psychiatric history rather than their current competence was the basis of job denials. "A couple of jobs I interviewed for," reported one man in our study, "I told them I was schizophrenic, and they just kinda made— well, that was the end of the interview." A woman with schizophrenia recalled: "A man who was recruiting me for a job called, and, when I told him [I had psychiatric problems] he got off the phone and he hasn't called me back." Another consumer reported: "I remember applying to a [fast food restaurant] . . . and I put down on there that I was a manic-depressive. And the manager started questioning me about it. 'Well, do you have a psychiatrist?' And I could tell once we started talking about it that I wasn't going to get the job. And I was overqualified for that job." Yet another of our respondents observed simply: "One prospective employer stopped the interview early when I disclosed mental illness. He was very rude."

Other consumers even had job offers taken back after disclosure of mental illness: "I applied for employment at a well-known national engineering company," recalled one person, "and received a job offering with the condition that I bring a work release note from my doctor. (The company knew that I had not been working due to an illness.) When I gave them the note stating that I was mentally ill but could now work, they discovered they could no longer afford to hire me." A man whose anxiety disorder produced limitations unrelated to the job for which he was applying nevertheless had the following experience:

I went in to a place that was located right next door to NAMI, and I gave the resume to this secretary. . . . I showed my portfolio [to the president of the company]. I was applying for a design, desktop publishing type position, and they said, "You've got a lot of experience in a lot of these different areas and you've got experience in communications and writing. Why haven't you been hired?" And I said, "Well, because I have an anxiety disorder, but it doesn't affect my ability to work. I just can't take the elevator above a certain floor or take public transportation." And there was that kind of visual change in the person. They were basically ready to give me an offer [and then it was] "Well, we'll get in touch with you." And then I never heard back from that.

Another reported similarly: "I was on a list waiting for a job. The job had been promised to me at the next opening. I never got the job when the supervisor learned I was a consumer."

Even clearer were occasional instances where consumers conducted experiments and found different outcomes depending upon disclosure of their mental health treatment history: "I was denied a job because I had circled the fact that I had psychiatric disorder. But then I reapplied again. . . . This time I did not put I was mentally ill or taking psychotropic medication. I got the job." Another put it quite simply: "After I got out of the mental hospital I soon found that nobody would hire a schizophrenic unless you lied."

Discriminatory treatment in the workplace also occurred when a person who was already employed developed a psychiatric disorder or when a disorder that had been concealed became known. As noted in chapter 5, a psychiatric diagnosis often causes others to view the person as less competent. To many employers less competent meant unable to handle the job, and knowledge of the employee's mental illness brought undesired and undeserved consequences. Some consumers were fired or asked to leave their jobs. "I worked in schools, as a school psychologist," reported one consumer. "I never told ahead of time [about my mental illness], but if hospitalized subsequently, there were often detrimental repercussions, such as being fired, or put on probation. I was once asked (by a supervisor with a master's in counseling), 'How do I know you won't hurt the children?'" A man with schizoaffective disorder had a similar experience with a school job: "When they found out that I had a mental background, they wouldn't let me work for the school district anymore. As soon as they found out I had any kind of mental disability, I lost my job." Another observed: "It's ironic that one work experience that I had as, of all things, a Health Planner, I was forced to resign from after my boss found out that I had a mental illness. . . . As soon as I told them I had schizophrenia, I think my boss asked for my resignation within a week. . . . And you would think they would have had some compassion, but they didn't."

On other occasions, working consumers were not fired outright or asked directly to resign, but were instead demoted and/or given jobs with less responsibility. "When I was first diagnosed," wrote one survey respondent, "I made the mistake of telling my supervisor at the time what was going on. She decided I couldn't handle a job I'd been doing for ten years and demoted me." A computer programmer described a similar situation: "After my most recent hospitalization for major depression, my situation at work has been difficult. . . . The assignments I was given were things meant to 'keep me busy' but were NOT typical analyst programmer tasks. Repeated requests for more work as well as more relevant (to my abilities) tasks were simply ignored [despite the fact that] both the quality and quantity of my work has been consistently high and is well documented."

Having a mental illness also led to limitations on advancement. "One former employer repeatedly refused to promote me in spite of my supervisor's consistent good evaluations," reported one consumer. "On one occasion I was told by the employer that I 'shouldn't tell people about that mental health shit' and that continuing to do so would prevent me from getting promoted anywhere." A man who had experienced depression talked about similar advice given in the military: "When I first went in [the Navy] . . . they make it a point that you never, ever want to say anything about depression or mental illness because once that is in your record, that is the kiss of death. You will never be promoted in pay grade or rank and you may as well just sign your papers and get out." "I have been denied promotions and even lateral movement within my workplace," said another survey respondent. "[Some coworkers and managers] have been very difficult to coexist with. Supposedly, I'm faking my illness to get out of work, not trying hard enough and the basic 'you're not qualified for management.' It's bad enough having schizophrenia without having salt rubbed in my wounds." A woman with major depression described the discouraging result of her hard work: "My attendance [at work] has been very good, missing only four days due to physical illness or scheduled medical tests—this in spite of another episode of major depression in the spring. . . . I maintained both the quantity and quality of work during this second bout of severe major depression, but it took a heavy personal toll and may have contributed to making my recovery more difficult. . . . In June I asked my boss just what it was going to take to get a promotion. My boss looked at me directly and said that I do not stand a chance of being promoted. While he did not say directly it was because of my mental illness, the implication was definitely there."

Those consumers who get or retain jobs may also face more subtle forms of discrimination involving violation of legal mandates that many employers do not fully understand and, hence, fail to fulfill. One requirement of disability law, for example, is that employers act so that the workplace is not a hostile environment for disabled workers. A work environment in which disabled persons are isolated, teased, or harassed does not provide them a true equal opportunity. Many respondents in our study reported that their work environments involved just these negatives and that they were sometimes driven from their jobs as a result. More than one in four survey respondents (29 percent) reported that coworkers or supervisors at work were seldom or never supportive or accommodating when they learned the person was a consumer.[5]

"You go from one day being a valued employee and everything is fine," said one woman interviewed, "and then I went on leave of absence and somehow they found out that I was in a psychiatric facility during that period of time and they were cold as ice. Everybody treated me different. They didn't even give me a chance. They wanted me out of there basically. They made it so miserable for me those last few months I was there, I had no choice but to leave. It was not a tolerable work environment for me. There was no more friendly conversation or chit chat. Nothing. None of the good things that you look forward to." Another survey respondent reported that he had been successful at getting a job as a corrections officer, but "at the first training session, we were asked to list any medications we took. I was then taking lithium. When they found that out they made my life so miserable that I took what I called a forced quit on their advice." A third noted painful social isolation at work as a consequence of disclosure: "This was the first time I openly admitted why I was absent (hospitalized for major depression). In the past I feared retaliation and repercussions, so I had not been open about my psychiatric illness. Upon my return to work, the first two months, only four coworkers would even speak to me."

One woman with bipolar disorder noted that such lack of acceptance of employees with psychiatric disorders occurred even in the mental health setting in which she was employed: "I was kind of fair game for those people who didn't really like working with consumers, who had that kind of prejudice. And I took a lot of heat that way in terms of being kind of a second-class employee—not by management as much, but by my peers, my coworkers. . . . There were some people who were very uncomfortable working around consumers and they would exaggerate any kind of mistake or they were always trying to make a case for why consumers shouldn't be in these positions." Her experience with mental health coworkers was similar to that of another consumer: "I now work in the mental health system where I live. Some clinical staff whose credentials are no greater than my own treat me with disrespect and suspicion. One union representative stood up at an employee meeting when I was first hired and said sarcastically that people 'should know he is consumer' before working with me." Yet a third lamented: "Not only have I found supervisors who were aware of my background not helpful (including psychiatrists), but rather they use the information against you when it is to their advantage. While a person who has a consumer history and [is] a professionally credentialed expert is an asset to any facility, it is usually viewed as a threat."

The Americans with Disabilities Act also calls for "reasonable accommodations" to permit disabled workers to continue on the job. What accommodations are "reasonable" is a matter of judgment (and often debate), but, for people with mental illnesses, such accommodations have included time off to attend doctor or therapist appointments, flexible work hours, and work space that is quieter or less visually distracting. Numerous consumers reported, however, that their employers and supervisors were unwilling to provide these types of accommodations. "I have had to leave a group therapy program I had been attending once a week for 1 1/2 hours," said one woman, "because of intolerance by my management to the regular absence from work, even though I regularly put in extra time to make up for that nonproductive time." Another woman with multiple psychiatric problems found that even her documented needs were not accommodated:

> [My psychiatrist] had written a letter to the company doctor. . . .
> He had asked that I be put in a sequestered work place, which is
> no problem because all I did was enter data in a computer at the
> time . . . and that I be given an understanding supervisor and time
> to go to these appointments with him. When I came back, I was
> not given a sequestered work place. I was told that they would
> appreciate it if I would go see the doctor at night and not on
> work hours. And I said, "The doctor doesn't work at night and
> not on work hours." And I said, "You may dock me for the pay.
> I will make up the time like I have before." This, of course, was
> leading to my layoff.

Still a third person reported that her requests for accommodations were not only denied but actually led to harsher treatment: "[At a job] I had to tell them that I had to see a therapist on a certain day and a doctor to get medication. And they said okay for a while, no problem. And then, for some reason . . . they says, 'Well, we can't do that for you anymore.' And I says, 'Well, let me know what day I can have off so I can schedule it.' 'Well, that ain't the way we work things.' I didn't think that was fair because a lot of people have a certain day off. But because I needed a specific time to go they knew why. They just didn't want to cooperate. . . . And eventually they started cutting my hours down to nothing. It seemed like they wanted me to quit."

Although such experiences were clearly too common, it is, once again, important to recognize that they were not universal. Some employers and coworkers were nondiscriminatory and highly accom-modating. One woman talked at length about her positive experiences: "I'm applying for a mental health job. And [a friend I had listed as a reference] got called and they started asking her questions and she said 'I'm so glad that you're thinking of hiring her because she's a great person even though she. . . ,'" and the lady said, 'What?' And she said, 'Well, her mental illness. You knew she was bipolar, right?' And she just kind of let the cat out of the bag right there. And the lady said, 'No, I didn't know that, but that won't affect it at all.'" The woman got the job and subsequently found her employers supportive and accommodating: "I've had instances where I've been in the hospital and I come out and just so my getting back to work runs smoothly, they'll give me a little extra time to get back into work." A man receiving treatment for depression described the similarly satisfying response he received from his employer when his mental illness became known: "I teach CPR on a part-time basis for several groups. I spoke to the director of the continuing education division, and I told her up front that I was being treated. . . . My evaluations were very high rated, so [the director] said, 'That's all that's required.' As long as I had good evaluations, then she had no problem with my mental illness problems that were under control with medication."

On rare occasions, consumers even found companies that were eager to hire consumers. Unfortunately, this was sometimes associated with a different form of discrimination—exploitation. "[The company I work for]," observed one of these consumers, "uses my illness to treat me badly and to their advantage. So they don't pay me as much as people doing the same job (although I am an expert and do a better job than they do) because I can't defend myself like regular people in communications [or] confrontations. And of course I have a label so they feel they can do whatever they want and treat me any way they want to." A similar dilemma was experienced by a woman working in graphic design:

My former employer seemed to hire only people with mental illnesses. . . . I don't know why the employer just hired these people. Probably just to take advantage of them 'cuz that's what he ended up doing. If people are labeled, other employers wouldn't employ them, and he could pay them less. And if he wanted to get rid of somebody, he would just use their illness against them. I was doing the same as people that make $16 to $17 an hour. And I did it better than they did, and I was more dependable. And it's hard to understand why these other people are making more than I am. . . . But they didn't want to pay me what they paid other people, and that was very frustrating. . . . They just plain said, 'we're not going to pay you any more than $7 an hour "cuz we don't have to."'

Another observed: "Instead of having a job that pays a decent living wage, I work part time as a clerk for $5.00 an hour. At one time I made in excess of $45,000 a year. However, since my 'illness' became known in my past industry, things have changed."

Paid employment was not the only place for discrimination to occur. Consumers also noted problems in trying either to obtain or to retain volunteer positions. As noted in chapter 4, many consumers who sought to contribute in the mental health field found themselves denied the opportunity, even as unpaid volunteers, to give to others for whose experience of psychiatric disorder they had particular sympathy; one in five consumers (20 percent) reported that they had sometimes, often, or very often experienced such denial. As one woman reported: "I tried to do volunteer work at a sheltered workshop. They said, 'We have standing policies that no clients, active clients or former clients up to five years after the fact, can volunteer.'" Another reported encountering similar exclusionary policies: "After I got my MSW, I wanted to volunteer at this one counseling clinic . . . and they would not let me volunteer because of my history, regardless of my therapeutic skills and credentials and education or whatever. They just said, 'No. You have a history of depression. You have a history of being unstable. We cannot allow you to volunteer here.'"

Not just the mental health field, however, denied consumers as volunteers. More than one out of every four of our survey respondents (26 percent) reported that they had sometimes, often, or very often been turned away from volunteer positions outside the mental health field when their consumer status was revealed.[6] "I had applied for some volunteer work at a sheriff's department taking reports over the phone on vandalism and theft," recounted one survey respondent. "On the application, it asked if I had ever been treated for mental illness and/or been in a psychiatric facility. I answered honestly, offering to provide references and allow them to consult with my doctor. Eventually, they called and said my background check came out okay. . . . I was supposed to let them know when I was available to work, which I did immediately. As it turned out, I never heard from them again. I believe it is because of my mental illness." Another consumer, a person with Tourette's disorder, reported similar lack of success trying to fill a volunteer position with a law enforcement agency: "There was another time I wanted to volunteer for the sheriff's department, just as a kind of thing where they just drive around and report things that went on. And they asked me what kind of medication you take and just because of my medication, they told me I failed their oral interview, because of the fact that they figured, 'Well, since he's on Prozac, then he must not be stable enough to go out there and just report when he sees someone doing something wrong.' They thought it was too overwhelming for me." Another consumer told this story: "I try to volunteer as much as I can, . . . but if it includes contact with kids or with other people directly, like regular groups like Red Cross or group homes, or even something that includes some connection with the group, I am not allowed to volunteer because something MIGHT happen." A similar message was given to a woman with dissociative and anxiety disorders: "I've been turned down for volunteer work because they don't want anybody with a mental illness being a volunteer for insurance reasons and stuff. 'Cuz something might happen. I don't know what, but something might happen."

One consumer told in even greater detail of the unreasonable and infuriating limitations she faced in trying to do good work for children:

I work as the Family and Community Involvement Coordinator for a small school district. . . . One of my jobs is to foster cooperative relationships between our schools and community organizations, businesses, and governmental units. In January of

1995, I learned about an excellent YMCA program called Young Leaders [which] helps develop the leadership skills of fourth and fifth graders. . . . Participating schools are required to supply two to four volunteer staff members for the camp. As the school district staff person who was responsible for getting our district's approval to participate in the Young Leaders Program . . . it was assumed by the YMCA staff and my district that I would be one of the camp volunteers. I was eager to comply. I have worked with young people in a variety of similar programs. In fact, I was the 1985 recipient of a prestigious award for organizing [the county] celebration of the United Nations International Youth Year. You cannot imagine my shock and anger when I reached the part on the volunteer staff application that reads: "Please note that volunteers who are being treated for any emotional or mental illness, including psychosis, depressive illness (depression and manic depression) will not be admitted. Experience has shown that this can be harmful to these youth and adults." I was angry, hurt, and troubled by how I was to handle this dilemma. I was the one who had brought this excellent program to my school district, and our participation necessitated my involvement as a volunteer staff member. We had a group of kids who were excited and ready to go to camp for three days. And I was banned because I would have a "harmful effect" on the kids and adults attending.

Although work—paid or volunteer—was the biggest focus of consumers' concern, discriminatory treatment in other aspects of their lives was noted also by consumers (in response to survey questions that specifically asked about such situations). Denial of housing on the basis of mental illness, for example, is also illegal; stereotype-based beliefs that prior psychiatric diagnosis or treatment makes a person a poor tenant are not acceptable grounds to deny that person a place to live. However, about one in five (19 percent) of our survey respondents reported that they had at least sometimes had difficulty renting an apartment or finding other housing when their status as a consumer was known,[7] an even higher rate than found by Bruce Link and his colleagues (10 percent) in their 1997 study.[8] "I have talked to some landlords," reported a man who has had depression, "and explained to them that I'm on a limited income and I do have mental health problems which are stabilized with medication. And once I state that, they don't want to talk to me anymore." Another recalled: "Three times [I was] denied rents because landlords knew my life history. One found out after I had moved my belongings into the apartment and made me move them back out or he would take them to the town dump himself." Still another told of the difficulty he had asserting his rights to federal housing: "The manager of the federally subsidized apartment complex where I have resided for nearly four years now didn't want to give me an application when I revealed that my disability was mental illness. She said she would mail me an application, but she didn't. I phoned her two or three times saying I hadn't received the application. She just said that she hadn't gotten around to mailing it. . . . It took a call from my therapist before she would send me an application. After I moved into my apartment, she made a point of telling me that there would be no problem if I wanted to move out on short notice."

A couple of consumers told how eviction from their homes was added to the stress of psychiatric hospitalization, leaving them with no place to live once they were discharged: "Once I was in an apartment and was evicted," reported one woman who now directs a mental health advocacy group. "They liked me a lot. I was quiet, and the place was immaculate. But I'd be in tennis clothes one day, and the next day I'd be in the hospital. And they were just frightened. So they evicted me when I was in the hospital. I couldn't believe it. I just was overwhelmed." Another said similarly: "I was evicted from my apartment while I was in crisis. It wasn't anything I said or did. I went to a mental hospital and [was] evicted while hospitalized (rent was paid). Landlord didn't want me there. I was discharged from the hospital and had to go to a shelter to live."

A smaller percentage of survey respondents (15 percent) reported having been denied educational opportunities. It is worth noting, again, that actual discrimination was difficult to establish. Educational institutions and programs are often highly selective and a fragmented course of education, whatever the cause, may be sufficient to make one less competitive with other applicants. Psychiatric impairments that interfere with one's ability to function successfully within an academic environment can lead to lower grades, conflict with instructors, or other problems that *are* legitimate reasons for dismissal from school. Nevertheless, in the opinion of some consumers, their illness—not their performance—was the cause of the inappropriate or discriminatory actions. Said one: "The head of the department told me that (even though I was an A student) she no longer wanted me in her program." Another reported that: "I was thrown out of a Ph.D. program . . . midway through by an advisor who had known about my illness since its onset several years earlier. . . . He made it clear that my illness was the reason." Some consumer comments, however, had more to do with what they were *told* by others about likely discrimination than with actual encounters with differential treatment. "I wanted to go to school," said one woman with depression, "[and was told] if you are a consumer you've got a problem that we can't take you in our school because you have a problem. They never know when I'm going to have a reaction or something." Another woman noted: "I had also been told the last time that I was in the hospital by another student that if I applied for the masters program if anybody would find out that I was a consumer, I would be removed from the program."

Matters even as routine as obtaining a driver's license were made more difficult by a history of psychiatric treatment, according to the reports of several consumers: "I am thirty-five years old and have never been the cause of an accident nor received a speeding ticket since I have been driving, [yet my state] still asks questions on license applications—'Have you ever been in a psychiatric hospital?'" "During my last hospitalization, nothing was said about my driver's license until I was ready to go home, and I was asked how I would get to my therapist. . . . I had to fight because they wanted to take away my license [even though] I've never had so much as a warning on my driving and, of course, no accidents." "About six years ago, I renewed my driver's license and I marked the 'mental illness' box. . . . Six months, no license until a board of six psychiatrists gave the ok." "Although I have not been denied a driver's license, the DMV requires my psychiatrist to fill out a form every six months or so, verifying that I am competent to drive."

One issue of discrimination that has received considerable attention in recent years is health insurance. Although severe and persistent mental illnesses are exactly the kind of health problems for which insurance is most needed—that is, problems for which the cost of care is enough to overwhelm almost any budget—many consumers found difficulty obtaining or retaining such coverage. Almost one in three (29 percent), for example, indicated that they had been turned down for health insurance, with their "preexisting" mental disorder the usual cause of denial.[9] "I went through a long period of getting jobs which offered health insurance," wrote one consumer, "but the health insurance had a preexisting condition clause written into it. It was standard for them to tell me I had to wait five years to get health coverage for mental illness. Of course, I'd be dead." "I had a lady [from the insurance company who] called me," said a young woman with bipolar disorder, "and [she] asked me a few questions and one of them was 'Have you been hospitalized lately?' And I had to tell her about being at a local psychiatric hospital. And as soon as she heard that she said, 'Okay, thank you,' and hung up. And then I got a letter in the mail that said they denied me coverage." Another consumer recalled the health insurance consequence of becoming unemployed: "I lost my job, and I lost my health insurance, . . . and there was an increased rate to keep it. I could keep it; they did offer it to me. But I would've had to pay more, plus the lifetime limit—there was a maximum of $25,000—had already been paid out. And then I tried four different companies and they would not insure me [because of a] preexisting condition." Still another reported a long and unsuccessful search for insurance: "I went to the library and did quite a bit of research on [insurance], and I probably investigated twenty-five companies and either called or inquired or learned through the literature that they would not consider anybody with a previous history of mental illness. And they did not bother to find out what your treatment history was. I wrote down that I had never been hospitalized and I have also never lost a job, nor have I ever been incarcerated for my mental illness, that I've been a productive member of society with a professional job for over twenty-five years, but that I needed to continue to get medication. That didn't make any difference. It seems that no matter, if you have previous history, you're not considered."

For consumers in these situations, they felt penalized for both their disorders and their honesty: "When I tried to apply for health insurance, two of the companies asked me if I had had a psychiatric hospitalization. And I responded with the truth. They told me that I could not receive medical insurance. So to receive medical insurance I had to lie. . . . I felt once again that I was victimized or being penalized for something that was, that I hadn't done anything wrong. But yet I had to lie, and I don't lie." Another person with schizo-affective disorder expressed her similar indignation: "Right now, with my company paid insurance, I have been turned down for my condition. I have to do without insurance until my company finds someone to take me. I don't have the same insurance that my coworkers have due to my illness. I feel I am being punished for being mentally ill. I work over forty hours, five days a week, and they said they can't give me insurance. No one will accept me."

Those who could obtain health insurance faced problems created by the nature and degree of coverage provided for mental illnesses. As mental health advocates have noted, one discriminatory aspect of most health insurance policies is the amount of coverage provided for mental health care: it is often substantially less than that for physical health problems and therefore inadequate to the needs of people with mental illnesses, particularly those with severe and persistent illnesses who may need multiple hospitalizations and long-term care. This failure of insurance companies to provide equal coverage for mental and physical illnesses created treatment dilemmas for many consumers. In particular, many consumers found themselves relegated to lower quality or reduced care; almost one in three of our survey respondents (31 percent) reported that they had sometimes, often, or very often been denied mental health treatment because of insufficiencies of health insurance coverage. "The insurance company gives forty-five inpatient days a year," reported one respondent. "And there's been times, where I could no longer go to the hospital anymore because I had used up the forty-five days. . . . There were times where I probably needed to be hospitalized but could not be because there was no insurance benefits left." Still another faced a similar situation: "Those twenty-eight days that I was in that mental health facility used up almost, probably within a thousand of the

$25,000 maximum that my policy allows me. In other words, when I got out of that facility, I only had probably less than a thousand dollars that would help cover any mental health services after that. So that quickly ran out, and I wound up . . . in a situation where either I had to quit going to see somebody or I would have to pay out of pocket."

Those who could not forgo treatment found themselves facing the added stress of overwhelming financial debt. "The major problem other than work problems," wrote one survey respondent, "has been health insurance discrimination. . . . My carrier had a one-million-dollar lifetime limit for nonpsychiatric illness and a fifty-thousand-dollar limit for psychiatric. I went through bankruptcy because of excessive medical bills." Another explained: "[In] April or May of 1996 I get a letter from the medical benefits coordinator of my wife's policy, and they tell me that they will not pay the second hospitalization because I've already reached the maximum $25,000 allowed under the policy—that's lifetime maximum. So that throws another fifteen or so thousand dollars onto my debt load."

Premature discharge from hospitals when insurance money ran out was also a concern of consumers in our study. "One thing I experienced when I was in the hospital," said one woman who had been treated for depression, "was watching people who were nowhere near being well and on morning rounds being told they had to leave the hospital that day because their insurance company had called and said they weren't covering any more. I was flabbergasted because I couldn't believe that these seriously unwell people were being put out to face incredible situations all over again when they weren't anywhere close to being well just because of the insurance or lack of it." Another sufferer of depression described the risk to her own life: "Things reached a low point, and I did attempt suicide. My benefits had run out by that time. So, although I had attempted suicide, I was in for a week, and it was decided I was better. I felt I needed to be in the hospital, and I couldn't be. . . . If I had had just about anything other than an emotional or a mental problem . . . I would still be covered. . . . I mean, I wanted to get out, because who likes being in the hospital, but I shouldn't have been out. I felt expendable. It was like your life is worth saving as long as you have money to back this up."

Moreover, not only inpatient expenses taxed pocketbooks. Still another concerned consumer talked angrily about the need to 'budget' outpatient therapy and the inequities between physical and mental health care:

> One of the areas that has affected me, almost every single year, has been the number of hours of outpatient therapy. . . . The hours have run out, and I can't afford . . . paying the full fee to a psychiatrist in order to be able to get treated. . . . I know by the first of September, I had eight hours left. I guess the thing that really makes me angry is what is the difference between seeing some psychiatrist and getting medication versus seeing an internal medicine doctor or your family practice doctor for everything else needing medication? And I know that I would have been a lot healthier through the month of December if I would have been able to see someone. And, in fact, I have made appointments to see my internal medicine doctor just to have that contact and say "Look, this really isn't working but I can't go to see a psychiatrist because I don't have enough hours." That doesn't make sense to me. The one thing I have to keep on top of all year long is how much time is being spent in trying to treat the illness. I don't know anyone else who sits and figures out all of that when they have heart disease or are diabetic or whatever, whether or not they've spent too much time in getting their illness treated.

Still another added this note of sarcasm: "When my insurance runs out for the year (usually by June), I am amazingly better, and they decide I only have to have therapy once a month the rest of the year. And I suddenly need more therapy more often when my insurance is beginning a new year."

More than one consumer reported being forced by financial need to get services at locales distant from both their homes and important sources of personal support. Said one: "I was sent to the state hospital rather than being treated locally where I could be with my family [because my insurance wouldn't pay for local treatment]. I was sent to [a city] which is 130 miles from where I live. . . . I didn't get to see my mom or my daughter. . . . [I felt] lonely, and mad that I couldn't be treated locally." Another reported similarly: "Because I didn't have insurance, I couldn't stay in the hospital. So they sent me to [another town]. Now I didn't like that at all 'cuz I didn't know anybody [there]. And I didn't want to be moved. I thought that was horrible. I didn't have a choice." Still another consumer observed simply: "If I had better insurance, I could pick and choose who I could see, and I probably would be better quicker."

Health insurance was not the only product inaccessible to those with psychiatric histories; consumers in our survey also reported problems obtaining life insurance. Those whose disorders had led them to despair and attempted suicide had particular difficulty finding insurers willing to take the risk that they would not return to a suicidal state. As one person explained: "I cannot get life insurance because of my past records. Because I tried suicide a couple of times and that's a big no-no. You can forget ever getting life insurance if you're mentally ill because you're a bad risk. So forget life insurance. And I've tried five different companies." Although the reluctance of life insurers to take on clients who have a demonstrated vulnerability to suicide is understandable (although suicide exclusion clauses could conceivably reduce the risk of issuing a policy even to these clients), coverage was also denied on the basis of mental illness even in the absence of suicidal history, according to the reports of consumers in our survey. One person, for instance, indicated: "I had a guy come and see me and when I told him that I had a mental illness . . . he just kinda went 'Well, our company won't cover you.'" "They refused to write a policy on me after they found out that I had mental illness," said another. A third described how: "I applied for life insurance, and I was denied. I'm sure it was because I was schizophrenic because other than that I'm in perfect health."

Even automobile insurance was more difficult to obtain with a psychiatric history: "I got a new car," reported one woman, "and I applied for some car insurance, and I made the mistake of telling the man that I suffered from depression. Well, he told me immediately that I would have to pay high insurance rates because, if I suffered from depression, I might get in the car and decide to drive at a high rate of speed and not only kill myself but take other people with me." Another consumer was given a different explanation for denial:

"When I applied [for car insurance], they asked about medications. They wanted to deny coverage because I took medication for depression and manic-depression even though my driving record was spotless for over eighteen years at the time."

Finally, a number of consumers felt that they were not protected by the law in the same way as people without mental illnesses. One in five survey respondents (20 percent), for example, reported that the fact that they were consumers was used against them in legal proceedings.[10] Child custody was one issue where a number of consumers reported being at a disadvantage. One woman stated: "I had my children taken away from me because the lawyer showed my psych record, and it was almost four inches thick. . . . So I feel as though they used my mental illness as a means to take my children away." Another woman, who had suffered from depression, wrote: "I am a loving, compassionate, faithful BUT noncustodial mom of two very wonderful children. . . . My exhusband is a successful and affluent attorney. Throughout our numerous and humiliating court hearings, he fabricated many, many lies concerning my so-called 'unstable' condition. . . . My psychiatrist and psychologist could attest to my sound mind and parenting skills, but my former husband did all in his power to refute their claims and discredit them. The stigma of mental illness was very prevalent here." Yet another woman reported that, following a hospitalization for major depression, she and her former husband

> . . . went to court several times over the course of a year in a custody battle. During that time, I remained stable, worked, and continued medication and therapy. . . . My doctor had testified on my behalf, stating that I should have the children and there was no reason why I shouldn't. As a parent, they had nothing on me except that my kids got too much fast food and soda pop when I was working and going to school at the same time. . . . [My exhusband] had a history of two DUI's [Driving Under the Influence charges], was arrested for possession of amphetamines, was arrested for possession of pot . . . and perjured himself twice on the stand. BUT, because I had a MENTAL ILLNESS and was treated in a psychiatric unit of a hospital, he was the better parent.

Consumers likewise had difficulty regaining custody, shared custody, or even full visitation privileges. "I never had a history of mental illness until 1994," wrote one woman, "following the 1992 Hurricane Andrew in Miami, my husband's loss of funding at the university, and our deteriorating marriage. Due to ensuing depression, I lost my children and am still awaiting overnight unsupervised with my children. Needless to say, for a professional who works with children and raised two boys, this was devastating. The court system operates in the Dark Ages." "I had more trouble in regaining custody of my children due to my mental illness," wrote another woman. "They told me that I had to stay out of the hospital for at least one year. It took me *five* years [out of the hospital] to gain custody." Still another reported: "I was in the state hospital when my exhusband died. My daughter's custody was turned over to an aunt on her father's side. It was never explained what my rights were, and I went years before finding out it was only temporary guardianship that was given." "My exwife had me institutionalized," said a man, "and then used the fact that I had been institutionalized as a justification to ask the divorce court to prevent me from having visitation rights and to restrict me from seeing my son until he was a teenager."

Psychiatric history was used to discredit consumers in other kinds of legal disputes as well, making it difficult for them to get justice for their claims. One consumer tearfully described how she (and her husband) had been unsuccessful recovering costs in court after automobile accidents: "They made me go for a deposition and they tore me apart, asking me about my mental illness. . . . And, even though these accidents were not my fault, we ended up not getting anything. Our case was dropped. Our cars were never completely covered and paid for by the other people. They just completely and totally got away with it." Describing another courtroom case concerning an automobile accident, a woman noted: "Because I was a mental health consumer who had the term 'lithium' written all over the medical records, a lawyer who represented the car insurance company basically stated that I was anything but a normal person."

Even for victims of serious crimes, mental illness made justice elusive. In fact, several people reported occasions when they did not even pursue criminal charges because they believed, or were advised, that their psychiatric history would give them no chance of success. One woman diagnosed with multiple personality disorder and depression, for instance, recounted the following: "Somebody that I knew wanted to talk to me about his wife who was getting really depressed. I said I would tell him what was helpful for me, . . . and we got together, and he raped me. And I talked to the district attorney, and I told her that I had this diagnosis. I said my concern was that my diagnosis would be either I was multiple and that one of my parts came out and asked for it or something equally sickening or I wasn't and, oh, what a nut. And she said yes, that would probably be the case. . . . And the thing is it feels like not having equal representation under the law because his crime wouldn't have been on trial. I would have been on trial." Another woman reported: "I was once raped in a date-rape situation. When I thought of pressing charges, a victim's advocate advised me not to when I told her I suffered from a mental illness. She felt it would be used against me in court." A third said similarly: "I was told by my therapist not to press sexual assault charges this year because I am a consumer." And one woman with bipolar disorder who did go to court discovered first-hand what the others had only feared: "My psychiatric history was admitted to court during a rape trial in which I was the victim/survivor." A similar dilemma was mentioned with respect to pursuing allegations of abuse or mistreatment by mental health caregivers. "I have had people in the mental health field and law enforcement ignore my claims of mistreatment by others," wrote one man, "once those others claimed that I was 'insane.' The mental health people and law enforcement people used my claims of mistreatment as evidence that I was 'paranoid.'"

The legal experiences described by consumers certainly contradict the popular perception sometimes expressed that people with mental illnesses are favored in the courts.[11] The notion that courts and laws are overly sympathetic to mental health consumers—for example, allowing them to escape the consequences of criminal behavior through insanity pleas—is largely unfounded. Not only are public beliefs about the use and outcome of insanity pleas incorrect,[12] but also any sympathy-fueled favoritism toward sufferers of mental illness that might exist in other kinds of proceedings seems greatly overshadowed by the instances in which the lack of credibility conferred by mental illness leads to unjust, even cruel, outcomes.

Consumer encounters with discrimination, then, appear frequent and varied. Their experiences once again verify that the negative attitudes toward mental illness revealed in earlier studies are indeed acted upon by those they encounter and that, however improved public understanding of mental illness may be, it has not spared consumers from continuing discrimination. On the contrary, consumers have found that their psychiatric diagnoses, their histories of psychiatric treatment, and their medication records inappropriately—and often illegally—disqualify them for many privileges granted to others. They have been denied jobs, demoted, or fired by employers when their status as mental health consumers was revealed. On the job, they have been neither given the accommodations mandated by law nor appropriately protected from stressful and/or hostile work environments resulting from the uninformed behavior of coworkers. They have been denied and discouraged from educational and volunteer opportunities, deprived of housing, and even had driving privileges questioned because of mental illness. As a result of discriminatory limitations on insurance coverage of mental health problems, consumers have sometimes done without needed care or been forced to accept lower quantity *and* quality of care. Even more devastating, they have lost custody of their children, and they have been unable to obtain legal redress or protection when victimized by others.

7

Indirect

Stigma

To this point, we have focused on experiences in which the reactions of others were directed at, or in response to, the individual consumer. Consumers reported how they themselves were shunned, avoided, patronized, discriminated against, and so on, when others found out about their illnesses. These are certainly fundamental examples of the ways those with psychiatric disorders are viewed and treated less favorably by others. A type of experience that is sometimes overlooked in its frequency and importance, however, is what I call "indirect stigma." With this term, I describe situations in which others are reacting or referring in negative ways not to the individual consumer but to other consumers or to consumers in general, and consumers witness or overhear these situations. When consumers recover and resume roles in the community, as is increasingly the case, they have greater opportunities for this type of indirect encounter of negative attitudes toward mental illness, as others who do not know that they have had psychiatric treatment or diagnosis feel free to express negative sentiments about mental illness in front of them. These types of experiences, in fact, were the most common kind of stigma experience reported by the consumers in our study. Almost 80 percent of our survey respondents, for instance, reported that they had at least sometimes been in situations where they had heard others say unfavorable or offensive things about consumers and their illnesses; half said they experienced this often or very often in their lives.

One type of experience involved hearing people disparage others by using psychiatric terms. For instance, one consumer reported: "I have been in situations where when someone did not indulge a person or asserted feelings contrary to that person's wishes, the incident was described by that person (scornfully) as a schizophrenia attack. Sadly, to be associated with schizophrenia is to be treated with less respect." Another indicated: "I've heard people say something like 'he's psychotic,' but they're saying it in a way to be funny—talking about people who aren't really mentally ill but who may not be acting the way they think they should be acting in a given situation."

Witnessing the common and careless use of slang terms for people with mental illnesses or for treatment facilities was also troubling to some consumers in our survey. Said one: "Ignorant people make slurs about 'goofballs' or 'that one didn't take his lithium.'" Another described people talking about someone's sister who had become ill and "saying over and over her sister had been berserk and wacko." "In casual conversation," said still another, "people will sometimes use the term wacko, crazy, nuts, those kinds of things that are terribly offensive about a person who has mental illness." One woman, who reported that she has become a collector of "mental illnessisms," noted that "there are more degrading [terms] about mental illness than for any other illness" and cited examples both domestic ("a little nuts," "he's a little loony," "one card short of a full deck," "she went off the deep end") and foreign ("there's too many kangaroos on his back field").

That such experiences are common should not surprise any of us. We need only to count the times that we have heard others (or perhaps ourselves) complain about "the lunatic" who designed the current tax forms or express anger toward the aggressive commuter "driving like a madman" or challenged ideas we thought were foolish by declaring that the one who offered them must be "out of his mind." And, in making those comments, we probably failed to consider that there might be consumers within earshot—perhaps friends or coworkers—who could be hurt or offended. Consumers in our survey let us know clearly that they were not only sensitive to such comments but also offended and hurt by them. To consumers, the message from these kinds of comments was clear: A psychiatric label is an insult, a disgrace, a source of ridicule, and, harking back again to Goffman, a feature that is thoroughly discrediting.[1]

The judgmental ways others talk about mental illness likewise communicates to listeners, including consumers, that mental illness is shameful and disreputable. Sometimes inflection and tone of voice—and the emphatic use of third person pronouns—communicate disapproval of those with mental illnesses: "When people come on the floor here [at work] who are getting treatment in the community, there's always a lot of giggling and poking fun," explained a social worker in our study. "I don't know why they take THOSE people everywhere. I don't know why they let THEM on this floor. Why do we have to put up with THEM?'" Another person reported: "I just recently was at a conference between forensics and the police. Some of the things they were saying, like 'those people.' . . . It was just a lot of stuff in poor taste." At other times, the very secretive or embarrassed manner in which people talk suggests a shameful aspect of mental illness: "I've worked for the government," explained one respondent, "and they always talk about counseling in hushed tones, like it's gossip."

Sometimes the disparaging messages are even clearer—and harsher. One consumer reported: "I heard teachers in my Catholic grade school say things like 'People in mental hospitals are so evil that it destroyed their minds' or 'If only people in Central Hospital would repent of their sins, they would be cured.' A priest in a sermon said about the mentally ill, 'sick people can't witness Christ, so if you are sick leave us and get cured.'" Another respondent recalled: "I was talking to a man the other day, and he said [that] Nixon let out all the crazy people in the 50s and that's why so much more violent activity is going on downtown." A third described a disheartening conversation with a neighbor: "There was a neighbor that grew up a block away, and there was another neighbor that grew up a couple blocks in the other direction. Well, I hadn't seen the one neighbor in a number of years, and we were talking about the old neighborhood. And he said he had just recently seen this one person and this person has had problems. He said he started to talk to him, but he got away from him as quick as he could because he's a loony. . . . He grew up with the kid, but he didn't even want to [talk to him]."

One man with an anxiety disorder found himself a witness and uncomfortable participant in behind-the-back (but in front of him) ridicule of a business client:

> The director of the art department had a client which was the Anxiety Disorders Association of America. . . . The director [of the Association] came down to the art department and was talking about the brochure that she wants to design of some sort. And when she left . . . the director started brainstorming about what are some things we can do for the design cover for her brochure? And then he started joking about, just making every kind of joke there could be about anxiety disorders. "Well, we could put Edvard Munch's *The Scream* on there, yuk, yuk, yuk." That kind of thing. I was laughing not because it was funny but because I don't want to be overly sensitive. But after the third or fourth time, I'm realizing . . . he knows I've got an anxiety disorder. . . . If I were black and somebody said "Let's put Little Black Sambo on the cover of this thing," nobody would laugh.

A man with schizoaffective disorder observed similar behind-the-back put-downs of another consumer: "There's a lady that goes to a place that I frequent, and oftentimes comments are made about her. . . . They call her Crazy Kathy and stuff like that. And the poor girl doesn't even know that they're talking about her because she tries to interact with them. And most of the people just kind of laugh up their sleeve at her."

Consumers in our survey were also witness to discrimination against other consumers and heard the comments made to justify that discrimination. They were in the audiences of community meetings when neighbors protested introducing group homes for people with mental illnesses or when politicians proposed screening voters with mental illness. They were in staff meetings where decisions to fire hospitalized colleagues were discussed. They fielded insults when they went out to increase opportunities for others with mental disorders: "We went up to the local community college," one consumer-advocate wrote, "trying to get the mentally ill considered to be part of the disabled student program. And the lady that was in charge of the disabled students—we were talking to her about the mentally ill and having a college program for people with psychological disabilities. She said, 'No, no, I wouldn't want that in the college. I worked with those mentally ill on my internship at a state hospital and they all smell the same, they have a certain odor.'" To this consumer's credit, she did not stomp angrily out of the office, but tried instead to educate the guardian of the disabled student program through her own example: "So we said to her, 'Well, do we smell?' She said, 'No, why should you?' And we said, 'Well, we're mentally ill.'"

Consumers also reported concern about how commonplace jokes about mental illness are. Whereas poking fun at other serious conditions—cancer, AIDS, multiple sclerosis, physical handicaps, and so on—are generally seen as in poor taste, humor about mental illness seems perfectly acceptable. One consumer reported: "I've heard people make jokes about mentally ill people. My mom was saying she heard a minister at church joke about consumers." Another described her reaction to such flippancy: "I see people all over [including, most recently at her son's wrestling match] with tee-shirts and whatnot that say 'Psycho' on them. It makes me want to tear it off. It isn't funny. It's not a joke." Still another person reported that her former supervisor, even though he knew that she suffered from bipolar disorder, brought the following humor column (which she enclosed in her survey response) to a staff meeting "and put that thing in front of me and the other staff":

Psychiatric Hotline

Hello. Welcome to the Psychiatric Hotline.

If you are obsessive-compulsive, please press 1 repeatedly.

If you are co-dependent, please ask someone to press 2.

If you have multiple personalities, please press 3, 4, 5, and 6.

If you are schizophrenic, listen carefully and a little voice will tell you which number to press.

If you are manic-depressive, it doesn't matter which number you press. No one will answer.

If you are paranoid, we know who you are and what you want. Just stay on the line so we can trace the call.

Consumers reported also being bothered by hearing psychiatric medications treated as a joke. "I'm a dental hygienist," reported a woman suffering from bipolar disorder [and probably taking lithium as part of her treatment], "and I heard a dentist say to an assistant just within the last month that she was manic and the dentist should give her some lithium. And it was a ribbing type joking way. . . . But it was a put-down type of comment and I was like 'Ouch!' You don't even know whose toes you are stepping on by saying that out loud." Another person with bipolar disorder remarked: "People joke about medication, and when somebody in a group is acting kind of wild one day, they joke and say, 'Have you taken your lithium today?' A manager [said this during a new staff orientation] and there was probably fifty or sixty people around. . . . And I thought to myself, 'You don't really know what you're talking about.'"

Although there is some difference of opinion among consumers about the acceptability of humor related to mental illness, most respondents seemed to consider mental illness itself no laughing matter. Humor such as one frequently hears was perceived as demonstrating a lack of appreciation for the consumers' experience and as communicating to them that they—and their painful conditions—are not taken seriously by others. Moreover, the obvious ridicule in much of this humor was hurtful. One can imagine how it feels to be in the position where, as one consumer observed sadly, "people make jokes to me all the time about me."

As recipients of mental health services, consumers are frequently in settings surrounded by mental health caregivers. They are often in a position, then, to witness interactions between those caregivers and the consumers in their programs. What they often witness, according to the reports of our survey participants, is not supportive, understanding care but rather harsh, unflattering remarks directed at other consumers around them or consumers in general. Sometimes respondents talked about overtly abusive behavior. "At [my treatment center] they call them stupid and crazy," noted one consumer, "and they talk loud to them and they talk like they don't understand that that person has got feelings like they do." This same respondent noted a specific instance that made a distinct impression on her: "This girl, she had a problem with her boyfriend. She thought that he really liked her, but everyone else was saying that she was really crazy. The other people thought, 'That crazy girl. You all better send her back to the state [hospital] and all that stuff. But I don't think they should have did it like that. . . . But they was calling her crazy and stupid, and that can hurt anybody's feelings. . . . I felt bad because I have had that same thing done to me." Another consumer reported that: "I've overheard things by other doctors about patients in the ER. They would say, 'Oh, she's just a routine psych patient.'"

Several consumers reported the experience of overhearing staff joking with one another about mental illness *in front of* or *within earshot of* those for whom they were providing care. "While this may fall more under the category of abuse in hospitals or lack of proper staff training," noted one of our respondents, "I feel these people [staff members] clearly demonstrated stigma against the patients through insensitivity to patients' needs, laughing about patients' behavior within their earshot." "As an outpatient," wrote another, "I have heard doctors talk and laugh about patients when they did not see me but others could hear them."

As noted previously, many of our consumer respondents worked or volunteered in mental health settings; many of these did so without disclosing their illnesses. These nondisclosures led to occasions when consumers were witness to humor at the expense of other consumers as well as unprofessional—and unethical—breaches of confidentiality. Said one woman: "I worked in a prison [where] a number of nurses would comment about the psych patients, as well as some of the psychiatrists would. [They] would tell funny stories about what happened in therapy. And while the psychiatrist didn't mention them by name, you knew who they were. And yeah, they were funny stories, I will say that, and I laughed along with the rest of them, but it left a bad taste in my mouth." Although staff may view their conversations, particularly their use of humor and their ability to laugh about what they encounter in their work to be a reasonable way to cope with what can be a stressful job, they seemed not to appreciate the effect that it has on those consumers within easy earshot. "I hear staff people making jokes about clients. I went through that for a long time. I would sit and I would listen. A lot of them would say, 'Oh, it's harmless venting,' but to me it was hurtful. . . . It scares me when I hear staff making jokes about clients, because I wonder, 'How can these people turn around and give quality service if they're not taking that client seriously?'"

Other times, the comments overheard went beyond mere humor to become complaints and derogation. One person explained: "Being in social work, a lot of the people that I worked with had a lot of clients that were mentally ill, and it was amazing to me hearing them talk about them in real nonprofessional ways—quite rude, just crude. I was hearing about my own supervisor once telling about her own mother who was manic-depressive and calling her names and telling everyone about it, which really bothered me a lot, and that's one of the reasons I was real uncomfortable telling anybody about myself." "I'm in the closet where I work, except for a few people," said another participant, "and [my coworkers] often get impatient with consumers, like someone is just being mean or someone's being lazy when it's not either of those things. . . . It's not so much that it's directed towards me, but just kind of toward consumers in general." Similar experiences were noted again and again by consumers working in the mental health field: "While I was working as a LPN [licensed practical nurse], it was not uncommon to hear other staff referring to patients who had a diagnosis of mental illness in derogatory ways, merely because of their diagnosis." "I am a MSW [masters in social work] myself, and was oftentimes irritated at the remarks made by fellow colleagues about certain diagnoses." "I have been in situations where I have heard others say unfavorable or offensive things about consumers and their illnesses. It especially bothers me when I hear fellow mental health professional workers do this. They say things like 'I don't like him/her (consumer); he is a borderline,' etc." "I have worked at [a psychiatric facility]. As with many other facilities in which I have worked, the patients are spoken about with disrespect, sometimes mocked, and often spoken to in shaming ways."

Some consumers reported also that derogatory remarks about mental illness and those who suffer from them came from educators and from participants in training programs for caregivers. Both future mental health caregivers *and those teaching them* showed disdain and disrespect for sufferers of psychiatric disorder. "I'm attending class right now," reported one woman, "and I sit there, and I listen to what the instructor's telling me about mental institutions and I just listen. I have to keep my mouth shut because one of the things he wrote on the board was that institutions protect society from mentally ill persons." Another man, one with a schizoaffective disorder such as was being discussed in class, reported: "I was going to community college and [the instructor in one class] said to me that he thought most people that were schizophrenic did things like go up in towers with a gun and shoot people. . . . [He also said] 'people with schizophrenia are usually dirty and don't bathe.' I felt really bad and kind of ashamed." Still another person, a woman with depression, noted: "In abnormal psychology a few weeks ago, my instructor was going over mood disorders, and he was on major depression. . . . And he said that it was a luxury, that depression was a luxury."

Such authoritative disparagement of mental illness was not confined to undergraduate programs. "Once we were on the wards in the third year of medical school," wrote one consumer. "The treatment of psych patients in all rotations was awful. They would laugh at them, poke fun at them on rounds, disbelieve any physical complaint they had. . . . The treatment of suicide attempts was the worst. They would tell them too bad they hadn't succeeded." Another noted: "At school the MD students often made fun of those with emotional difficulties. In med. classes, the professors often told jokes and put-downs. Acronyms, such as 'GOMER' (Get Out of My Emergency Room), were taught. . . . My classmates would joke in front of me about antipsychotics, loony tunes, etc. . . . It hurt, but I told myself that they do not understand."

Consumers did not even have to leave their homes to encounter negative messages about themselves. They needed only to do what most Americans spend many hours a day doing in their own living rooms and kitchens and bedrooms—reading, viewing, and listening to mass media. More than three-quarters (77 percent) of the survey respondents reported that they had seen or read things in the mass media (e.g., television, movies, books) about consumers and their illnesses that they found hurtful or offensive. Almost half (47 percent) indicated that this occurred often or very often, while only one in five (22 percent) reported that witnessing hurtful depictions of mental illness occurred seldom or never.[2]

Many consumers reported being troubled by the general inaccuracy and exaggeration of media depictions. "I think like on TV they have to make it dramatic," noted one of our interviewees. "So they make it look more dramatic than being mentally ill really is."[3] As another interviewee observed: "There's a tendency to report the sensational, the well-known person that had obsessive-compulsive disorder who had just hordes and hordes of things in his house and never left his home and he had let his fingernails grow to enormous lengths—Howard Hughes. And just a tendency to portray the most extreme cases. . . . Or the Unabomber or serial killers or serial rapists. These are extreme examples of people with mental illnesses completely out of control." TV talk shows were said also to sensationalize psychiatric disorder and to present consumers in ways that made them seem more disturbed and out of control than is usual. "There are some programs, some of the talk shows, that make us look like jokes," said one woman we interviewed. "I've seen this thing on there that they had people who had multiple personality disorder. They made them look like a three ring circus. They made them look like freaks." Still another lamented: "I get really upset when I see the way they portray people with mental illness in movies and stuff because there's just not anyone who's positive. There's not anyone who shows any propensity toward leading a normal life."

Among the objections to media inaccuracy was concern about the misuse of legitimate psychiatric terms. Misuse of the word "schizophrenic" to mean divided or contrasting, in particular, was a sensitive point for consumers. As one person noted: "Well-respected, well-written magazines like *Newsweek* and *U.S. News and World Report* still a lot of times use the word 'schizophrenic' incorrectly. They use it in the sense of dichotomy." Reporters frequently describe unstable economies, shifting political positions, diverse cities, and even inconsistent sports teams as "schizophrenic."[4] Another consumer was sensitive to an advertising misuse: "There was this one company. They said, 'Our mixer is schizophrenic' because it had so many attachments that came with it. It could change from one appliance to another." A third reported: "There was this article in *PC Magazine* describing the action of a chip as being schizophrenic and able to act in many different ways. I thought that's inappropriate."

Misrepresentation of treatments was also noted: "I've had sixty-six electroconvulsive therapy treatments. It was nothing like what was . . . in [*One Flew Over the Cuckoo's Nest*] where Jack Nicholson was just writhing on the table, and it looked like a terribly inhumane kind of therapy. . . . And it had an enormous impact on me . . . just very, very frightening."

Consumers were also offended by the disrespect shown in media depictions and discussions of mental illness. Sometimes this was associated with radio and TV talk shows in which hosts or guests expressed negative sentiments about people with mental illnesses. Rush Limbaugh was identified by one of our interviewees as one of the people "who've said we're sponging off the government with our entitlements and our benefits and that we should go back to work." This consumer also went on to observe: "Psychiatry is not spoken about very highly on radio or television or politics. They consider people with mental illness not worthy to live in America. They hate the fact that we're getting free money from the government that we're entitled to. They want to take away our food stamps. They want us to starve. . . . Who are they to say whether or not I have morals or I'm lazy because I have mental illness, all people with mental illness are lazy? It bothers me." Another respondent was troubled by columnist George Will's attack on the Americans with Disabilities Act and his reported suggestions that "these people with mental problems, they were just troublemakers and difficult and really weren't disabled. They could straighten up and fly right if they wanted to." Still another person found the approach of religious shows to mental illness troubling: "What really galls me is the way religion on TV treats it. They're going to slap you on the head, be healed. And that I find offensive. They talk about mental illness like it was demons." "I have been offended by articles I have encountered in magazines and newspapers," wrote another survey respondent, "articles which, trying to be encouraging, downplay mental illness to nothing but a character flaw which can be simply overcome. All you have to do is 'put your mind to it.' Or else encourage you to 'turn it over to the Lord,' as if you are choosing to be depressed." "In the newspaper and even in flyers," observed still another consumer, "it's just that the mentally ill are always a burden to the rest of society."

Another aspect of concern was the use of disrespectful language. "You hear radio talk shows saying 'that nut job,' 'that crazy person,'" noted one of our interviewees. "They call psychiatrists 'shrinks.' Any reference to mental illness, they're going to have a derogatory slang expression for." Another said similarly: "On TV, certain programs say this person is crazy, this one's wacky and a real nut case. . . . They use certain phrases such as 'nut case,' 'wacky,' and 'crazy' that's upsetting to you. . . . I just cringe. I think, my gosh, they don't really know what this is all about and to use those kinds of words is really derogatory." Still another interviewee described an article in a university newspaper: "The title of it was 'It must be fun to be crazy,' where words like crazy and just kind of real inflammatory words were used. 'Cuckoos' and stuff like that." "I think that people's language in general is stigmatizing," was another consumer's observation. "You know, use the word 'crazy' and 'you're nuts' or 'you belong in the funny farm' and all those kinds of things. I see this pretty often in advertising and just in the media in general. I think the language that's used, I don't think people understand how pejorative it is towards people who have a serious mental illness."

Although television, films, and newspapers were the most often mentioned media sources, the most modern of information sources, the internet, was not without its contributions to stigmatizing depictions of mental illness. Consumers surf the web, just as others do, often in search of information about their disorders, and while they found some useful information, they also encountered offensive and stigmatizing references there: "Like on the internet," noted one man we interviewed, "newsgroups and stuff, you can see where if somebody doesn't say something that everybody likes, they label him crazy and they brand him with being schizophrenic or this and that." "I just heard about a site that's very derogatory for mental illness on the internet," reported another of our interviewees. "It's an interactive game with other internet users. You're supposed to survive in a fictitious state hospital as a mental patient. The staff gets more points for how many times you put the patient in seclusion or in restraints or give them forced medication and stuff like that. And the patient gets so many points taken off their score when they act out." A woman with dissociative identity disorder noted troubling information on the internet about her disorder: "I see a lot of stuff on the web, in the newsgroups; it's not exactly positive in regards to people with mental health problems. Like people with dissociative disorders are possessed by the devil and need to find God in order to be cured." A sufferer of Tourette's disorder commented about his use of the web to find information: "All you have to do is type in 'Tourette's Syndrome' and they have good things on there, but then they have people that kind of make fun and joke about it. . . . You have some people that treat it like we're almost demon possessed. And they kind of make fun of the fact that we have tics, and tics become a laughing matter. It becomes a big joke."

Advertising that featured insensitive exploitation of terms and images related to mental illness was included in consumer comments as well. For example, one survey participant noted: "There was this little hot dog shop . . . and it was like 'come in and have a hot dog to keep yourself out of Butner' and Butner is where there's another psychiatric hospital. That was just very cold. [Going to a hospital is] not something to make fun of. It's a very serious and difficult situation." Several people objected to a Sprint ad with Candace Bergen on a couch "telling her doctor that she was hearing voices telling her to switch to Sprint." Another recalled "some clothing agency in New York that said something about 'no more straitjackets' and had somebody in a straitjacket advertising a suit." "We received in-the-mail advertising," said one woman. "The outside of the envelope had on there 'Do you want to go crazy? Guaranteed to drive you crazy.' [It was] a promotion for starting to get videotapes of The Three Stooges. And in the whole letter, every paragraph had something involved 'you'll go nuts over this.' . . . and 'This will drive you crazy.' I was really really angry." Another woman who had had depression reported: "I was in a card shop one time, and they had a jar of nuts and the label was referring to the mentally ill. And they thought that was real cute. I was not impressed. To degrade someone who doesn't have a choice in the matter that badly as if it's a big joke really irritates me." Similar irritation was expressed by a male respondent describing a billboard ad for a "psycho" cola: "It's offensive because they're making money at the pain and suffering of other people."

Consumers also expressed dissatisfaction with other forms of media humor at the expense of people with mental illness. This included jokes and comedy sketches poking fun at mental illness: "Some movies I'm kind of offended by that portray people with mental illness as funny or nut cases," said one interviewee. Another indicated: "I know on comedy shows that mental health is always an object of comedy. And when you're living it, it's not. . . . There's television shows where the comedy is supposed to come because someone is out of touch with reality or crazy. They lend to that whole atmosphere of that people who may have any kind of use for mental health, whether it be medication or counseling, they're wide open to being the butt of jokes. And I don't appreciate that. . . . I just know that when somebody on TV starts making jokes about like schizophrenia where people hear voices and stuff, I just feel like, you know, this is no laughing matter." A third noted that, on Comedy Central, "they constantly make fun of people that are mentally ill," while a fourth gave this brief assessment of TV images of mental illness: "Portraying consumers as like fools. Mostly portraying them as idiots." Several consumers mentioned a comedy skit on *MAD TV* that they found particularly troublesome. In this skit, there was a game of 'Schizophrenic Jeopardy,' with the following elements, according to one interviewee: "The answers would all be like 'I do what the voices in my head tell me.' . . . and at the end even the one gal crawled across the floor and was . . . biting at the announcer's leg; she was growling and snarling."

As with overheard remarks, some consumers observed that ridicule of mental illness often came in the form of jokes about the medications they take to maintain their stability: the frequent implication is that such medications are indulgences used inappropriately just to manage everyday moods. "I found some buttons from this store," noted a woman with depression, "that said 'Have you taken your Prozac today?' And other similar things like 'Don't talk to me today. I haven't taken any Prozac yet.' Recently, in one of our local papers, there was a comic strip that showed a bunch of cubicles at work with IV bags that said 'Prozac,' and that's how they keep their employees at work."

Not all consumers were offended by this humor. Divergent views were also expressed. A few consumers felt that humor was positive, and they even used it themselves to deal with their illness and their feelings about illness. One survey participant reported that he has worked up a comedy routine based on his illness and performs it at holiday parties; he felt that the ability both to laugh at his illness and to be appreciated by others for his humor was therapeutic. Another consumer was even stronger in his endorsement of humor: "I don't think that fighting stigma is going around jumping on people who make a humor or joke about it. . . . In fact, humor is one of the most important coping skills that I've had in my life to fight this illness or disorder. . . . It takes the sting out of the seriousness that I feel, and it helps me through. One of my favorite jokes, from *The Far Side*, which has helped me through many a suicidal episode . . . is a man falling through the air calling on his cellular phone. He's saying, 'Hello. Suicide Hotline? I've changed my mind.' I would hate to see this type of humor squelched, but I know there is someone out there that would be offended by it. I still have the joke right next to my computer."

With their many complaints about the language and humor over-heard in social situations or media sources, in fact, consumers could be (and have been) accused of being overly sensitive and humorless. Some might even charge them with excessive political correctness and unnecessary enrollment in the "language police" for their reactions to "meaningless" jokes and phrases offered as entertaining, not intended to harm or offend. Consumers themselves even considered the possibility that they might be offended too easily, and they were certainly aware that others might view them as too thin-skinned or intolerant. One consumer, for example, after indicating that he had often seen or heard offensive things in the media, added "but I have a low threshold of what I find offensive." However, consumer reactions hardly seemed a blind devotion to political correctness. Their expressions of concern presented more a personal, emotional reaction to perceived ridicule than an espousal of a political position. In most instances cited, consumers indicated that they did nothing to insist on more "correct" behavior. In fact, they were often quite forgiving, by reminding themselves that the people responsible were simply careless or uninformed about mental illness: "Perhaps," suggested one woman, "people are not aware of how devastating this can be to someone; unless they've had personal experience, they may not realize the effects of the stigma." Another reasoned: "I don't think people realize, when they say stuff like that, they think that they're in a certain company, and they think that there's not anyone who could be sensitive to the issue in this company." A third was even more generously understanding: "In a way they probably don't intend to offend anyone because I'm sure the people that use those terms aren't people who realize what mental illness is. And I know that before I became closely involved with it . . . I wouldn't have been concerned about using a term saying, 'well, they're really crazy or nuts.'"

Moreover, consumers seemed not to desire inhibition of careless speech and inaccurate images about mental illness through insistence on established rules of social conduct but to reduce such language and images in recognition of the hurt it causes to those being ridiculed. As one man put it: "One of the fears I have is that we don't become another angry minority group and that people stop saying the remarks that they do because they don't want to be politically incorrect, but they really are able to assimilate a compassionate attitude for the situation and develop an attitude based on 'They're right; I understand what they're talking about.'"

Consumers did not seem to be objecting solely to what they saw and heard based upon principles or dogma. But they were aware that they were both troubled—hurt, offended, embarrassed, insulted—by what they witnessed and discouraged that these reference to and depictions of mental illness continued unfavorable public attitudes toward people like themselves. Often the inaccuracy identified related to the specific disorder with which the respondent had been diagnosed; then they very clearly saw the comments and depictions aimed at themselves. One interviewee with bipolar disorder, for instance, recalled a memo sent from a counselor at a community college where she was teaching: "It was a cartoon [that] showed a psychiatrist's office. And it had stairs to the upper level and the bottom door said 'depressed' and the top level said 'manic.' And she thought this was funny enough to send to hundreds of people." Another interviewee with the same disorder noted this inaccuracy: "Some of these made-for-TV movies, they misrepresent the mentally ill. Like somebody that's bipolar, they'll have them being schizophrenic at the same time." A third person with bipolar disorder commented that: "The word manic is used in the media often, usually in a negative manner, very commonly as a joke," adding, "for some of us, it's not a joke." Yet another recalled "a comic strip where it said 'manic depressive crossing.' And it was supposed to be funny. . . . I found it offensive." All four had been sensitized to these occurrences by their own diagnoses of bipolar disorder. Similarly, complaints about the depiction of multiple personality disorder came from a person diagnosed with that disorder: "Programs will show . . . my disorder, multiple personality disorder . . . on the talk shows; they'll make it an exhibition. These people will call out their personalities. And they can be cruel. I can remember seeing it on *Geraldo* once, and they made a joke out of it." A woman with borderline personality disorder reported that she "took offense personally" when, during a break in an educational seminar, "people were talking about people with borderline and what monsters they are and they are so difficult and so forth."

Moreover, the concerns were not only personal but also practical; people worried about how others who saw these inaccurate depictions viewed them as a result. As one person observed about a movie with a character with bipolar disorder: "It just didn't show a true picture of someone that really has the disorder. . . . It gives people that are not informed the wrong idea, and so it reinforces their fear. . . . They'd use that movie as a reference as to how someone that's manic-depressive acts or the symptoms that they experience and the things that could happen with someone that has that disorder."

The personal concern about what others would learn from inaccurate media depictions was made even clearer by a consumer with depression whose possible treatment included electroconvulsive therapy (ECT):

Last season on *Chicago Hope* they had a manic-depressive psychiatrist. . . . It was really accurate up until the point where they admitted her and gave her electroconvulsive therapy. And that was completely wrong. It's not the way they do it at all. They didn't even anesthetize her. They had her writhing. And that is not done. And that gives this horrific image of ECT. . . . It made it look like medieval torture. . . . And I think that's really harmful because it makes it that much more difficult for someone to ever admit that they have actually had that. It adds a huge amount of stigma to the psychiatrists who actually use the treatment. I remember when they had that scene on *Chicago Hope*, I think I called half my family. . . . This was only within a year of when I almost had ECT because I went treatment resistant and basically ran through every medication and needed something else. It was something that really, really frightened my sister that I might have this ECT. . . . And for me to think that she was watching the show and seeing it portrayed like this, and then the fact that some day I probably will wind up getting this. I just didn't want her to have that picture in mind when she thought of me.

Another consumer told of her fears upon seeing a TV movie depicting her disorder: "They portrayed someone with manic-depression, just portrayed her terribly. She was accused of some crime or something, . . . and they just made her out to be a wacko crazy person. And they never got to the point where they said this can be controlled with medicine or anything like that. . . . I had just gotten done telling my in-laws that I was manic-depressive, something which I kept from them for a long time . . . and then I see this on TV and I'm like, 'Aw, shit!' I had just told them and I'm like 'God, I hope they're not watching this.'" A third consumer saw media depictions as contributing to the isolation she experienced: "Entertainment movies . . . just really give the name of mental health a really bad picture. A lot of people haven't been in psychiatric units and they look at these movies and they say, 'Well, if that's the way those places are, I'm not going there.' I guess maybe the reason I'm so sensitive about it is because my family will not come visit me when I'm in the hospital."

The most common complaint of consumers about media depictions, however, was not about disrespect or humor, but concerned the association of mental illness with violence and criminality. Consumers noted, for example, the frequent depiction of persons with mental illness as violent villains in entertainment media. "You see stuff like that on TV all day long," observed one interviewee. "They make the mentally ill look like we're insane, that we need to be locked behind doors. It shows that people that are paranoid schizophrenic are dangerous, they're criminally-minded, they could kill you." "A lot of movies," noted another, "they'll start like 'Can this particular character avoid a psychotic killer before he gets too close?'" Many others expressed the same concerns: "Television portrays us as the villain all the time. You never see a good show where mentally ill people are highlighted as positive reinforcement. It's always negative things, where they are going in with an axe and they're killing everybody." "Sometimes in the movies and the media, they do portray people that have mental illness as being kind of scary, that we like to have chainsaws and cut people up and do that kind of stuff."

Another aspect of consumer concerns was about the harsh solutions suggested by psycho-killer films: "I have seen movies in which the 'psycho' villains are killed at the ending," observed one person, "and the audience is left with the feeling that the world is better without any 'psychos.'" Another man said: "I used to go to movie theaters quite often. . . . When there has been a tragic thing to happen, like a serial rapist or a murderer, or a pervert of some type, it seems like that person is kinda labeled along with it as a schizophrenic or a paranoid, or some type of mental illness. And it seems to me in most of the ones I've seen, the way it ends up is this person getting killed and mutilated or massacred in some great way. As if that person is no better than a dog. Like in the movies, where people are hunted down like animals and killed in some tragic way in the end."

Similar concern was expressed about frequent news stories involving criminal actions committed by people with psychiatric diagnoses where psychiatric status implicitly explained the criminal or violent behavior, thereby lending "factual" support to the entertainment images of 'psychotic killers.' "I think what bothers me most," said one interviewee, "is when you pick up a paper and you see there some guy has committed a crime and gone on a killing spree, they do not fail to mention this person has been depressed, has been under the care of some therapist, or hospitalized for a mental condition. Like as if that is his reason for doing what he is doing." "They bring up the fact that somebody killed people," noted another respondent, "and they blame it on the illness. They overemphasize the fact that the person's labeled with a certain illness." "Pretty much, on the news, we're violent," observed still another. "And they sensational-ize things, like on accidents and shootings. They might say 'This person has mental illness,' but they never say, 'Well, this person had cancer and that's why he killed.'" A fourth put it quite simply: "As far as the media go, only a story about a violent schizophrenic will do."

Consumers were likewise concerned that such crime stories with mentally ill perpetrators not only appeared often but also tended to remain a focus of attention for many days. One consumer, for ex-ample, cited a specific story in which "this guy who was mentally ill who was not seeing a doctor or getting counseling went in and shot two people about an argument over money. So for five days, for five long days, each day the local paper had a piece about him being men-tally ill."

These news stories, according to consumer respondents, also tended to show little sympathy or understanding for the person with mental illness in the story; the features did not consider other fac-tors—such as inadequate treatment resources—that may have con-tributed to the tragic outcome. One articulate consumer reported on this oversight.

I think it was *Inside Edition*. They were doing a profile of Wendall Williamson, who is a young man in North Carolina who was very psychotic who was, I think, abusing substances at the time. He was under the care of a psychiatrist. He was going to law school at University of North Carolina at Chapel Hill, and he had a break and he killed another student and wounded several other people. . . . And the way they portrayed him in the story was without any compassion towards him or understanding to-wards him. He's going to be in a psychiatric hospital for the rest of his life. . . . And then on *Inside Edition*, they certainly did not talk about anything that happened prior to that, that he had had some problems on campus; he had gotten thrown out of a bar once. He had altercations with the police once. So I think there were a lot of people who knew that he wasn't functioning well, but no one interceded until it was too late. And it didn't include that there might be remorse on his part or regret or that this was someone who obviously was in a great deal of pain a long time.

Similar sentiments about lack of compassion and misplaced emphasis were echoed by another consumer: "We read that this is what you can expect out of the mentally ill. And you may read that they have been for mental health treatment. But you don't read the news media saying where the mental health treatment may have failed. Or where the public may have failed by not putting enough funding or seeing about the mentally ill well enough to avoid some of these things. The news media blames it on the persons with mental illness."

Of course, consumers' central concern is that these stories and images convince the public that those with psychiatric disorders are characteristically violent and dangerous, despite the research evidence (noted previously) that demonstrates consistently that the vast majority of people with psychiatric disorders are neither violent nor criminal.[5] "This man went berserk and killed a couple of nuns some time ago," noted one of our interviewees, "and it was always pointed out that he was mentally ill. This may be true. This may be a fact. But the fact that it was pointed out that he was mentally ill is a reflection on all people that suffer from mental illness. It says that all of them are capable of doing something like that to the public. . . . But this happens over and over and over again that heinous crimes are associated with mental illness." Another observed: "The good things that consumers do and have done are overlooked, and the media tends to concentrate on the sensational bad things that people do. . . . And the public doesn't seem to know the difference. So they get a lot of these images that people who have mental illness are all crazed criminals, and they can't be trusted around anybody's children or they can't be trusted period."

Still another concerned consumer noted: "Most of the time [in the media], it's some fictionalized portrayal of a person that's an axe murderer, just a very dangerous person that you can set them off at the drop of a hat. If you say the wrong thing, they might blow up in your face. . . . People get the preconceived notion that everybody is dangerous if they've got a problem." "They'll take a situation where a bad crime is committed by someone with a mental illness, and they'll capitalize on that. And then people that see these things on television or read it in papers, if they don't have any mental illness in their own family, it gives them the wrong message." A woman with depression commented similarly: "I do not like to see 'former mental patient' or 'mental patient' when violent acts have been committed. This seems to perpetuate fear that we are dangerous." And a man with schizophrenia expressed concern that "when a psychopathic killer or someone like Jeffrey Dahmer or a post office worker that came in and shot a bunch of coworkers—when the media reveal this type of person is a paranoid schizophrenic (and that's my diagnosis) . . . that makes me kind of regretful that that kind of stuff has to be publicized so much when it's really the exception and not the rule." Another person observed: "[The media] only cover the very worst case outcomes—you know, postal employee runs into post office, the main branch. He shoots up a bunch of people. . . . These are the things that are, for lack of a better word, glamorized. The result is that people automatically seem to make this huge leap from 'this person has some problems and they are trying to do what they can with them' [and] automatically it goes to 'watch out because they could be the next one to invade the office and kill a bunch of people.'"

Once again, the concerns were not simply for accuracy but also for potential personal consequences of such portrayals: "It seems like the newspapers, if they can, find a link to psych," observed one of our interviewees. "And then they crack down at the state hospitals and at the psych wards because somebody did a crime. . . . It makes all psych survivors look like they're criminals." Another noted that news stories about crimes committed by people with psychiatric illnesses "is where my in-laws got the idea 'Oh, God, how awful. No baby while I am around them.'"

Consumer observations about the prevalence of news and entertainment depictions of people with mental illnesses as violent and dangerous have been borne out in numerous research studies, as noted in chapter 2. Most commonly a mentally ill character in prime-time television is the villain.[6] More than 70 percent of the major characters with mental illness in prime-time drama are violent.[7] News stories about crimes committed by a person with mental illness are more likely to appear than other stories about mental illness and more likely to get front-page space and sensationalized headlines than stories about other crimes.[8] Consumers are, therefore, not imagining the common media connection of mental illness and violence. Beyond what other research has already revealed about the nature of media depictions of dangerousness, our study results tell us that consumers are both very much aware of such depictions and sensitive to and troubled by those depictions. Such portrayals do not pass unnoticed, and they affect those who see them and take them personally. So powerful are these depictions in communicating the dangerousness of people with psychiatric disorder, in fact, that one respondent described the self-doubts arising from his encounters with such stories: "Every time I either read or watch what a dangerous, killing person I am supposed to be, I used to get scared. Could I do that? I don't think they—the media—would get by with it if it wasn't true."

Stigmatizing portrayals in the media are unquestionably common. However, it would be unfair to overlook that fact that mass media also occasionally provide accurate, informative, and sympathetic presentations about mental illness. These too were noted—and appreciated—by our consumer respondents. Several people mentioned positive coverage, in both the print and broadcast media, when Margot Kidder went public about her bipolar disorder in May 1996. Another noted the appearance of Mike Wallace, who has suffered from depression, on *Larry King Live* as an example of a "constructive" media presentation. One woman described what she felt was a positive article in her local paper: "Our paper printed a really good article because Theresa McGovern died here, and so there's a big article about that 'cuz they opened up the Theresa McGovern Treatment Center. . . . It told about her struggle and was actually a very good article that was realistic, that explained the struggle and basically that it could happen to anybody, it didn't matter if you were rich or poor."

These occasional encounters with positive portrayals of mental illness,[9] however, do not change the fact that almost all consumers in our survey had nevertheless encountered indirect stigma, many of them with great frequency. Almost all had been in positions to hear disparaging remarks, slang references, and jokes referring to people like themselves, that is, those with mental illnesses. Almost all had been witness to hurtful, offensive, and misleading messages about mental illness from almost all types of media, from radio to TV to newspapers to the internet. And that means that even those who may avoid discrimination or retain the support of their friends and family are unlikely to be spared the indirect stigma that pervades our conversations and our media.

8

Impact of

Stigma

One can imagine what it must be like for people to have the experiences described in previous chapters—to be shunned by friends and family, to be discriminated against by landlords and employers, to hear and see themselves depicted in disparaging and disrespectful ways. But we do not have to merely imagine. Once again, consumers can and did tell us directly how these experiences affected them. A number of consumers, for example, described their reactions in written remarks on the survey questionnaires, some of which have been revealed in the quoted comments in previous chapters. In addition, to be sure that we would learn about the impact of stigma experiences, we specifically asked each of our one hundred interviewees about their reactions and responses to each situation they described to us and recorded and tallied the specific reactions conveyed.[1] Results, as one would expect, revealed a variety of responses to stigma experiences.

Consumer responses indicated that stigma and discrimination experiences aroused strong emotions. A third (33) of our interviewees, for instance, described being angered and offended by what they encountered. "I feel angry," said one consumer. "I feel, we're in the 90s now and people should be well educated on this kind of thing. And I feel a lot of anger about it." In fact, anger, for some, was an understatement; terms like "furious" and "enraged" were not uncommon. One person said about overhearing negative comments about mental illness: "I felt as if I wanted to hit someone, I got so angry."

Almost as many interviewees (28) reported feeling hurt. They were wounded by what others said about them. One person, for example, described her reactions to comments in her church about weak faith being at the root of suicide: "It's hurtful. It's really painful. It's like, how could you think of me in that way?" Another interviewee described this reaction to overhearing joking stories about psychiatric patients: "[I was] sick at heart. I know for a fact that they don't tell funny stories about people with cancer or even at the time with people with AIDS . . . but somehow, because they were psych patients, they were more [acceptable] somehow. And that hurt, that really did." Still another told of the following incident: "I was in a thrift store once a couple of years ago, and I started having a panic attack. My hands felt clammy, and my heart started racing, and I guess my face flushed. And there was a woman one aisle over with her little girl and she said to her little girl, 'Come here, close to me. She's crazy.' [Then] she hustled her child off down the aisle really fast. . . . And it really broke my heart, it just broke my heart to hear a mother tell her daughter, the next generation, 'stay away from that person, she's crazy.'"

Consumers also reported feeling discouragement, disappointment, and frustration at the obstacles that public attitudes and discrimination seemed to present for them. "I was so disappointed," said one woman about comments on the job. "It's like, well, this is my life now, working with people who are intolerant." Some of those interviewed also talked about their sense of humiliation, embarrassment, and degradation. Speaking about media portrayals of mental illness, one person revealed that "it makes me feel like I should be ashamed of my illness." Furthermore, consumers reported emotions that mirrored or added to the symptoms already associated with their disorders. Eighteen of the interviewees, for example, explicitly indicated that they felt depression or sadness as a result of their experiences; three talked about their increased sense of helplessness. One person with diagnosed depression, for example, talked about her reaction to disrespectful treatment by health care professionals: "I just felt like the end of the world. I just felt so down and just suicidal. . . . It just keeps the illness going."

Of course, emotions are not simple, and they tend not to occur neatly and separately; thus a count of individual emotions reported may not do justice to the depth and complexity of possible reactions. This was certainly the case with the consumers in our study. Both on paper and in interviews the consumers reported reactions that offered a complex mix of many emotions. One woman, for instance, reported: "[I feel] really angry and hurt that in some way I'm defective as a human being because of something that I was just borned with. . . . And it really hurts, and I'm really angry about this whole thing. That I had to live my life like this and didn't get more support from other people." Another described how: "When I was turned down for a nursing job, [I felt] very angry and ashamed and isolated. It was like I was dirty and wasn't good enough to be with the rest of the people that were there. . . . I had to sit [in my car] for a few minutes because it does hurt, trying to pull your emotions back together again and questioning yourself. 'Why does this have to happen? Why can't people accept you as a human being as you are? Just because I have an illness, does that mean I'm contaminated?'"

Despite their intense feelings, most consumers did not voice them. They believed that they would not be listened to or that their emotional displays would just be taken as evidence of their "mental instability." "I know it's really vain," said one woman about her experiences of being treated as less competent than others, "but sometimes I want to say, 'My IQ is 158, what's yours? I'm not really a moron, so don't treat me like one. I think people would just see that as more hostility on the part of the crazy person. . . . If you confront anybody about anything, it's 'Oh, you always were more emotional.'" Consumers who had not disclosed their illnesses to others also worried that responding to hurtful or offensive remarks would expose them as consumers and open them up to more direct rejection and ridicule. "I had still made the decision to nondisclose," said one consumer who had overheard joking remarks about other consumers and explained that laughing along with them "was much easier than calling attention to myself." In addition, consumers sometimes felt that their expressions of concern or objection would be futile, would make no difference in what is an overwhelming pattern of negative attitudes among the vast majority of those they encounter. As one consumer put it, explaining why she did not say anything to people

making joking comments about mental illness: "I feel like I'm pushing against masses." Said another: "I don't really do anything. I just
don't like it. . . . There's nothing I can do about it."

Consumers, who often could not express their pain or outrage,
were forced either to suppress their feelings or to suffer them alone
and in isolation. "It makes me furious [hearing what people say about
consumers]," observed one interviewee, "but furious in a very sad
way. I don't act upon that. I'm just more likely to sit and feel pain for
a little while." Another said similarly, about comments overheard at
church: "I basically sat there and hurt. When I would get home or in
privacy, I might even cry about it. But I would not say anything."
Consumers, both to escape aversive situations and to prevent themselves from expressing feelings that might be poorly received and
misunderstood by others, might go off by themselves, thereby increasing both their sense of isolation and their actual distance from
others. "I kind of walk off on them," explained one woman with
bipolar disorder. "I just turn and walk out, that's how I handle a situation. And then I get very depressed and upset and I don't want to be
around people." Another described her similar reactions to coworkers' comments: "I just felt really bad, and it made me really depressed,
and I isolated a lot."

The effect of stigma and discrimination experiences went beyond
immediate emotions, however. Of our interviewees, when asked, 95
percent said that they believed their experiences had had lasting impact. They reported, for instance, that such experiences changed the
way they viewed and interacted with others. More than one-quarter
(27) of our interviewees reported that they had become less trusting
of others and more guarded in their interpersonal relationships as a
result of their encounters with negative public attitudes and discrimination. A sufferer of bipolar disorder explained: "I think I'm a little
bit more cautious about people. I used to believe and trust people a
lot more, and I know that I'm a lot less believing of them." Another
interviewee said simply, "I don't trust people as much." Still another
confessed to her interviewer: "I don't trust anybody anymore. I mean,
it's hard even talking to you." When the stigmatizing remarks or
discriminatory behavior came from mental health caregivers, they
undermined the very trust that is essential to successful therapeutic

work: "They've made me real distrustful for a long time of professionals," said one man. Another consumer, in response to the concluding survey question about possible willingness to be interviewed, added this to the end: "P.S.: I frankly don't trust mental health professionals. That's why I won't be interviewed by you!"

Because of their stigma experiences and their resultant distrust of others, many consumers have become reluctant to disclose their psychiatric illnesses to others. Of survey respondents, 74 percent indicated that they had avoided telling others outside their immediate family that they are consumers; almost half (47 percent) said they did this often or very often. "There's only one time I told someone about my condition," explained a woman with bipolar disorder, "and, because of that situation back-firing on me, I'm actually kind of scared doing it again. I'm just totally cautious about it because it just seems like I've had too many times where people have thought poorly about me even though they've worked with me a couple of years. And then, all of a sudden, it's like I tell them something like this, and they don't even see me the same way. It's scary. It's really scary. It's a big risk to take, to tell someone."

This sentiment—that it is too risky to reveal psychiatric history—was probably the most repeated one among our interviewees. Again and again, they told us of their reluctance to reveal their status as mental health consumers. Typical remarks from consumers included the following: "*I never reveal.* . . . Only a few special friends know my secret." "I used to feel I had to tell people about my illness but not any more. Not after some of the reactions I got." "I know that I used to be a fairly open person. Never, ever again. . . . I don't believe that anybody is going to be understanding any more." "Upon my return to work, telling my coworkers about my mental illness was not a consideration. Hiding it was. . . . I didn't have the strength to defend myself against any prejudices they might have."

A related impact of stigma noted by our survey participants was that it required them to become less honest. To protect themselves against rejection and discrimination, many had learned to answer questions about their psychiatric history falsely. In fact, 71 percent reported that they at least sometimes dishonestly avoided indicating their consumer status on written applications for fear that the information would be used against them; more than half (56 percent) said they did this often or very often. "I *never* reveal my illness (chronic depression)," said one person, "and have always lied about it for all applications, including insurance, military applications, and Peace Corps applications." "For a long time," said another, "I wouldn't say, or, in fact, I still won't say it on job applications because I realize that in the real work world a lot of people just don't understand." "On the question that concerns driver's licenses, there was a question of have you ever been treated for a mental illness," wrote still another consumer. "I checked no. I was lying, and I know I should not have. Although I am perfectly capable of driving a car and I am a safe driver, I felt that being truthful would prevent me from getting a license." A fourth confessed likewise that "I've routinely lied about my medical history when renewing my driver's license."

Such dishonesty, however, was often distasteful and at odds with the way consumers wanted to be; feelings of guilt, self-dissatisfaction, and anger at being forced into such dishonesty followed. "When I filled out applications afterward looking for work," explained one woman with whom we talked, "I never put down that I had been seen. . . . I felt rotten because I tend to be a moral person and do not lie. And that felt real terrible to me, and I was real guilty about it for quite a while. And then I just realized, well, that's what I'm going to have to do in order to survive. I had to compromise my ideals in order to get a job, and I did not feel good about it. And still don't." Another consumer who confessed to lying on applications described how "lying like that haunted me and exacerbated my fears and paranoia." Hiding psychiatric history also contributed to feelings of shame. Such secrecy or outright lying, after all, is what one does to protect a personal or family embarrassment. If it must be concealed, then it must be shameful. As one survey participant explained: "I have been able to hide [my status as consumer], which is helpful in such circumstances, but makes for all the more a sense of shame accompanying my trying to hide it."

Consumers also reported that their stigma experiences had led them to become more socially isolated. One way to avoid disclosure was to avoid contact with people who might perceive or find out about their illnesses. Almost one-third (31) of our interviewees said that one long-term effect of stigma was that they avoided social contact. "I used to want to be with people," said a man with schizophrenia. "Now I want to stay away from people." Another said simply: "I keep myself inside my yard because I figure I'm not welcome outside the yard." Other consumers limited their social circles to those they thought might be more understanding by virtue of their similar psychiatric backgrounds—other consumers. "I tried to protect myself from being found out," wrote a survey respondent, "by not having normal friends, or, if I did not know other mentally ill people my age, by not having friends at all for years at a time." Said another: "Now I tend to just have friends with the opposite sex that also have mental illnesses. It tends to be that my friends also have mental illnesses."

Those who did pursue friendships found that having a secret that they could not share with others—their mental illness—created barriers to social interaction. "It's harder to pursue friendships at work," explained one woman, "because you can't tell them about something that's part of you." "[Mental illness] means that I can never remarry," observed another. "It inhibits your ability to form relationships with other people. It absolutely prevents it." Still another noted: "It is more difficult to reach out and try to start new friendships, join a group. That part is definitely a barrier in my life just because it's a lack of trust of other people."

Stigma and discrimination experiences also lowered people's motivation to seek out other opportunities, such as jobs. One in five interviewees (21) said that they were now less likely to apply for jobs, schools, and so on because of their previous unsuccessful and painful experiences. Some feared another rejection. "Remembering some of the things that have happened before," said one person, "makes me not even put effort to even try to do some of the things that I want to do or wanted to do. . . . Not wanting to experience rejection . . . just made me not try at all." The discouragement they experienced as an immediate reaction to lack of success became, for some, a chronic pessimism about the future that destroyed their motivation. One woman listed all the many stigma elements that have decreased her motivation to do more and increased her desire to do less:

I feel hard to get enthusiastic about finding a new job or anything because either they treat you different or they don't promote you or you get less wages just because you have a mental illness. And if they don't find out about it, well, it makes it harder for yourself because occasionally you have to go to therapy and you have to schedule around the work hours. And therapists don't necessarily do that. So sometimes you have to go at the end of a work time. And of course, if you did that too much, an employer might catch on. Of course, he'll know because of insurance. If you file insurance to pay for it, they'll find out even if you don't tell them that you have a mental illness. And besides that, with computers nowadays, anybody looking to hire you or anything can just look up your social security number and it shows everything right there. . . . Here I am at home on social security disability.

Still others found themselves trapped in unsatisfying situations because of fears that attempted change might require disclosure (or additional disclosure) of their mental illness, with unknown results. One consumer, for example, explained: "I'm afraid to leave my existing job because I'll have to fill in those applications like that again, and who's going to hire me? So I feel like I kind of am stuck in a dead-end job." Another commented that her prior experiences "made me more wary about going out and looking for another job. I'd like to move from this very conservative area, and I'm hesitant to do that because I do have a job here. No telling what I'd be moving into."

Keeping one's psychiatric background a secret was burdensome in other ways, as well. For some, it was uncomfortable keeping secrets from others: "I think not being able to feel comfortable telling people about who I am [is one result of stigma]," explained one consumer. "And it is hurtful for not being able to share with other people. I would love it if I could just tell the people I work with and other people that I meet that I'm this way right away without having to worry about how they're going to take it." Concealment, as noted before, also increased consumers' sense of isolation: "I feel like I can't be totally candid with most people," said an interviewee. "Like I have a secret that I can't share. So it makes me feel kind of alone—

feel alone. And somewhat inferior." The need to conceal also contributed to consumers' anger and frustration. "I feel angry that I always have to be hiding, hiding," said one woman, "because it's not something I'm really ashamed of, but I just don't want to hear the crappy comments and put-downs."

Perhaps the greatest problem, however, was the substantial burden of anxiety experienced by consumers who lived under a constant fear that others might find out about their psychiatric status and respond unfavorably to them. The vast majority (79 percent) of our survey respondents reported worry that others would view them unfavorably because of their consumer status if they found out. More than half (56 percent) said they worried about this often or very often. "I always feel somewhat apprehensive," said one consumer, "about telling yet another person or having it brought out in another way. I just don't know how people are going to react." "I pride myself on my work," said another, "and I'm doing okay, but I'm still afraid that somehow the company that I'm working for is going to find out. . . . I have this awful feeling that somebody is going to find out about my past. And it's just going to ruin everything. I kind of live with that fear all the time." "I just don't tell anybody. . . . It scares me because I'm afraid they're going to find out, and then they can fire me for not being honest or for lying on the application. . . . And so I lie and I pray a lot."

For others the fear was even more intense. "I remember being terrified," wrote one survey participant, "for anyone to find out that I had been hospitalized with a suicidal depression after the birth of my child. I felt sure that they would reject me and label me." Another stated similarly strong fears: "I am virtually petrified of revealing that I have a mental illness and have been hospitalized, especially since I work in the field of psychology." A third spoke of a mixture of both fear and anger: "I get angry because I'm living a secret life," she said. "The people where I work and a lot of the people I socialize with don't know that I've had these problems. And I live in fear of them finding out because I know that they will treat me differently."

Moreover, concealing mental illness is not a simple matter of keeping silent. Concealment requires great effort and vigilance, according to the consumers who spoke and wrote to us. "I feel that I always have to be on guard," said woman with bipolar disorder. "I try very, very hard—and have been fairly successful—in keeping this knowledge from people and circumstances that could use it to hurt me. But I'm always wary. I'm always thinking, 'Boy, I'm really down today, but, boy, I better not let anybody know.'" A consumer working as a psychiatric nurse explained how her secret complicated her life: "Where I practice therapy, no one knows there. And that makes it really hard because right now I've had a lot of problems. I was started on a [new medication], and I've had a lot of problems with the medication, and yet I'm not at liberty to say anything. And then, you always have the problem, have I told this person or has it been this one over here. It gets to feel like you're walking a tightrope."

People sometimes went to great lengths (and added to their own stress) to keep others from finding out. "I live in fear of [people] finding out," explained one person suffering from depression. "That's one of the reasons why I drive thirty miles away from my home to go see my psychiatrist. It kinda keeps it kinda distant, and you kind of reduce the chances of running into people." Another described how, to keep her "high-powered job" despite multiple hospitalizations, she "always had to tell them fibs like mastectomies and aunts that didn't exist had died." One person even denied herself successful treatments to avoid any possibility of disclosure of her bipolar disorder: "When I learned I was gonna get the job as patient advocate, I cut down my lithium . . . because I didn't want to have hand tremors at work . . . because I feel that if my hands are shaking, people know there's something wrong with me. And so—this is how bad stigma is—I cut down [my dosage], and within four months I was in a full-fledged manic episode and lost my job. . . . I denied myself my medication and I hurt myself because I wanted to be just like everybody else and not have any telltale signs about me that I might be on medication. I didn't want to lose credibility. That's how bad stigma can get."

Bruce Link and his colleagues have provided empirical evidence that the burdens imposed by concealment of psychiatric history has deleterious effects. In a 1991 study with more than five hundred individuals diagnosed with major depression or schizophrenia, they found that attempts to maintain secrecy were largely ineffective in reducing the psychological distress and demoralization associated with stigma. In fact, they concluded that "secrecy is associated with a shift towards worse outcome in terms of demoralization."[2]

An additional impact of stigma experiences was reluctance to seek needed treatment. About one in ten interviewees (11) said that their experiences had made them less likely to pursue professional help. Messages that they were lacking in character or will or faith, for example, kept them from treatment. "Because of stigma," said one consumer, "I have really fought going into the hospital repeatedly. . . . And, by the time I ended up in the hospital, I was in pretty bad shape." Disrespect from mental health caregivers also discouraged help seeking. "It's made me cautious," said an interviewee. "It's made me more selective. I won't be so eager to go see anybody because of the experiences I've had with the psychiatric community."

Consumers were not unaware of how some of these responses might appear to others, including (or perhaps, especially) mental health professionals. They recognized that increased distrust could be easily interpreted by others as merely a manifestation of their disorders rather than an understandable result of their stigma experiences. "I think I'm a more cautious, less naive person now," confessed one interviewee with schizophrenia, who added, "Some people would even say paranoid." Likewise, consumers were aware that their increased isolation and avoidance of social contact could be seen as "social withdrawal," a symptom of illnesses such as schizophrenia and manic-depression. Their reluctance to pursue jobs and school could be perceived, if not as "laziness," by the general population, then, by clinicians, as "apathy" symptomatic of their disorders.

Others reported that their reactions did indeed involve clinically intense and prolonged symptoms. The increase in problematic emotions such as depression, for instance, was, for some, not merely an immediate and short-lived effect of their stigma experiences, but a long-term consequence fueled by rejection, discouragement, isolation, and loss of opportunities. Fourteen of our one hundred interviewees stated clearly that they felt their experiences had had a long-term effect in prolonging such symptoms. As one person with depression described it: "If you were depressed before, try isolating yourself and people avoiding you and that kind of stuff. It just makes you more and more depressed."

The most common long-term results of stigma described by consumers, however, were lowered self-esteem and self-confidence; fifty-seven of our one hundred interviewees, as well as many other survey respondents, mentioned this decline. "It's affected my self-esteem to the point that a lot of the time I even have to question my own decisions on stuff I do," said a consumer with bipolar disorder. "It only takes for them to make one critical remark, and it's kind of like I plummet. . . . I get so low that I can't even do my housework." Jokes and disrespect and messages about lacking competence, such as consumers repeatedly encountered, led to what many observers have called "internalized" stigma. Consumers constantly take in and accept unfavorable views about mental health consumers; eventually they view themselves in similarly negative ways. "After a while," said one interviewee, "when people continuously [shun you], somehow can make you almost believe that you're not as good as they are. It makes you feel bad, and that's how I felt." Consumers repeatedly voiced such sentiments about internalized stigma: "I fight the stigma, and then I buy into it. I'm not as good a person. There must be something wrong with me. I must not deserve better." "If nobody's willing to give you a chance, you start thinking, 'Well, maybe I don't deserve the chance.' There's no way you can totally not internalize some of what you get from the outside if it's repeatedly the same feedback." "When you're told either verbally or nonverbally that you are not good and not as good as others, it starts to sink in after a while, especially when your defenses are down in the first place because of low self-esteem. I think my self-esteem has really suffered because of the way I've been treated. And that's something that's not easily fixed."

Stigma experiences, in fact, did not just have negative effects on self-esteem; they produced powerful and devastating effects, according to many consumers, which led them, as one survey respondent wrote, to "devaluing me, my life, my worth, and my talents." "You don't feel like you had anything to offer the world," observed another. "You were a freeloader, you were living off taxpayers, you were good-for-nothing. . . . You feel like you're stupid, that you have nothing to offer." And this person was hardly alone; others have had to overcome similarly harsh thoughts about themselves: "It made me feel like I must be some kind of freak, that I was nothing, that I had no opportunity to ever hope that there would be any kind of way that I would come back to be somewhere as you could call normal." "It makes you feel so guilty, like you shouldn't be on the face of the earth with this condition. And a lot of times it felt that way, you know, what am I here for?" "Since I experienced my illness, I know that deep down (as well as on top) I'm a piece of garbage, no self-esteem, that no one could possibly love me, etc." So powerful were the pervasive negative public attitudes that one consumer was even led to confess: "I am very ashamed of myself and what a waste of a human being I am."

Implicit in consumers' description of the results of their stigma and discrimination experiences is that stigma itself becomes a major barrier to their recovery. In making this assertion, I want to make clear that I am talking about the modern concept of recovery that goes beyond mere symptom reduction and hospital discharge as treatment goals; true recovery involves more than just symptom relief. As consumers, advocates, and mental health professionals have pointed out, recovery involves also a return to productive and satisfying lives just as can be expected by people recovering from physical disorders.[3] Those with mental illnesses wish for and strive for such recovery no less than people with other medical disorders. However, the stigma and discrimination they encounter does much to undermine such recovery.

It is hard, for example, to regain or maintain emotional stability when encounters with others hurt, frustrate, and anger, as consumers described. When the rejection and discrimination experiences so often witnessed or encountered foster distrust and sadness, as consumers reported, symptoms of paranoia and depression are that much more difficult to overcome. When emotional and interpersonal support—so important to all of us in weathering the crises of living—is lacking, as consumers so often found it to be, and when the stresses of rejection, insult, worry about disclosure, and guilt about deception are added to the burden of illness, recovery becomes a much harder task. And when opportunities that people need to be comfortable, contributing, motivated, and self-valuing members of the community—jobs, housing, education—are denied, full recovery is also denied.

"When you're mentally ill," noted one survey participant, "it's as though every prospect, real and potential, drops, drops, drops from sight. You're not seen as someone who needs a little more cushion, but as someone you wouldn't want to waste *any* cushion on."

Patricia Deegan—psychologist, consumer, and outspoken advocate for empowerment of mental health consumers—has described even more powerfully the impact of others' views on self-esteem and recovery:

> Finally, there is the stigma and the prescribed role of learned helplessness and patienthood that we have had to endure. It seems that we were systematically told that we could never follow our dreams and hopes and really become real people who live in the real world. Rather we were consistently told to avoid stress and to learn to cope . . . [and] the stigma and despairing messages did not stay in our environments. Slowly we internalized all the stigma and despair that surrounded us. We came to believe that we were as useless and as helpless and as hopeless as we were being treated. We learned to settle for less and less and actually began to believe that was all we could be. And this was the dangerous part. It was like a darkness began to settle over our hearts. The flame of hope and of dignity began to fade under the dark shadow of oppression. It was a type of dying: the death of hope, the death of dreams, the death of our humanness and our individuality.[4]

In contrast to these grim consequences of stigma, however, consumers were sometimes able to find positive results of their experiences. When asked about the impact of stigma experiences, one in ten of our interviewees indicated that they felt their experiences had helped them to become more compassionate and understanding of all people with disabilities. "I think, in a way," said one interviewee, "it's made me a more sensitive person to the needs of others and other mentally ill people." "It's made me a lot more tolerant of individuals who have mental health problems," said another. "I sure look at it in a different way." One person, who now works in the mental health field, felt that her own stigma experiences conferred greater ability to be empathic with her mental health clients: "I think it makes me a damn better therapist. . . . I think I can come from a unique perspective when I'm counseling my clients. . . . I think that they sense a sense of understanding from me that they might not get from somebody else who hasn't had the history. So that's a plus." Another consumer, however, described the mixed feelings associated with this growth in understanding: "There's no doubt in my mind that it's contributed to many positive aspects of my character. I really do understand what people go through. . . . I know what it's like to feel like there's talent within you that doesn't have the resources, the area, the place to make it come out. . . . [Although] for all the character building of the adversity that I've been through, I'm not so sure it wouldn't have been the opposite way. I would have liked to have tried the other way."

One in ten of our interviewees also suggested that they had been strengthened by their encounters with stigma: they had been toughened, made better equipped to endure, and become more confident that they could indeed survive whatever further hardships and mistreatment they might face. "I think I'm a stronger person now than I was two years ago," observed one interviewee. "So something good must have come out of this." "I think I've become tougher," said another. "I think I can handle adversity." A third explained: "[My self-esteem] is probably better because I know now that I'm a survivor and there's not much I can't handle."

Consumers also reported that they felt their stigma experiences may have increased their determination to learn more about their disorders and to overcome both their disorders and others' attitudes. Said one interviewee: "It has given me a drive to find answers that I know there are no answers to. . . . I've been trying to learn how to empower myself . . . and to help others in a way." A woman battling depression explained: "I feel like I gotta fight harder than the average person. It actually made me want to work harder to prove them wrong. And so, in some ways . . . it made me more determined."

Interviewees spoke of becoming more determined also to speak out and more committed to trying to combat stigma. A number believed that their involvement in mental health jobs and/or in advocacy groups devoted to fighting stigma had been fueled by their own personal experiences of stigma. "They make me more of an advocate for people who don't know as much about the system as I do," declared one person. Another described how stigma "motivated me to make it better. . . . I channel my frustrations into trying to make the system better." A third indicated that, because of her stigma experiences, "I've ended up becoming a very vocal mental health advocate. I've been teaching in community education classes, being involved with the local NAMI organization, doing Circle of Friends programs—just involved in speaking out and trying to educate people." Moreover, the motivation provided to attack stigma was quite powerful, in line with the intense feelings of hurt and anger described previously. More than one consumer participant used the term "mission" to describe their efforts. "I feel driven to do the work that I'm doing with CURE [a nonprofit organization to empower persons with mental and physical disabilities] because I think it's so important," said one such consumer. "So I've kind of turned this personal misfortune into a mission." "It has affected my life to such an extent," said another, "that I have committed my life to change that situation—both financially and emotionally become a missionary. . . . All our finances, past, present, and future, all my emotions and energies, past, present, and future [are committed] to this cause of changing stigma and discrimination against people with mental illness by society and professionals."

What consumers have told us, then, is that their stigma experiences have had significant impact on them, in both short and long terms. Their immediate effect aroused many negative emotions—hurt, frustration, discouragement, and especially anger. Their lasting negative effects include low self-esteem, social isolation, anxiety about disclosure, stressful efforts to conceal, and prolongation of symptoms like depression and distrust. All combine with discriminatory denial of opportunity to lower quality of life and impede recovery. It was remarkable, however, that many consumers were also able to see positives in the outcomes of their stigma experiences; to them they attributed increased empathic understanding of others, increased determination to recover, improved confidence in their ability to withstand travail, and stengthened motivation to become involved in mental health and advocacy work.

9

Strategies

and Coping

The recovery model that is growing in influence in the mental health field reminds us that we need to think about the strengths and resources of afflicted individuals rather than to focus exclusively on deficits and hardships. It urges us to remember that those with psychiatric disorders are not merely passive victims of their diseases; instead, they can be (and many are) active managers, searching for and trying out strategies to lessen the impact of adverse circumstances and finding ways to move ahead with their lives despite the obstacles they face.[1] Moreover, as Agnes Hatfield, a longtime mental health advocate and a founder of the National Alliance for the Mentally Ill, observed in a 1994 issue of the *Journal of the California Alliance for the Mentally Ill*, "it is important that those who support or treat people with mental illnesses become aware of the coping strategies that an individual uses."[2] Knowledge of such coping strategies not only aids understanding, but it also provides people, particularly those forced to cope with mental illnesses, better ideas of how they can help themselves and others.

Part of coping with mental illness is coping with both the stigma and discrimination that accompany it. In addition to finding out from consumers what their experiences of stigma and discrimination were, we wanted to learn more about how they coped with such experiences. Thus, in our interviews, we included a direct question about coping. We asked all one hundred interviewees: "What have you done to deal with the stigma of mental illness? What strategies have been helpful to you?" Their responses were sometimes saddening, sometimes inspiring, and at all times enlightening.

As consumer reports in the previous chapter indicated, many consumers utilized concealment as a strategy to protect themselves from stigma and discrimination. They were cautious as to whom they revealed their illnesses. They did not reveal their psychiatric history on applications for jobs, licenses, schools, volunteer organizations, and so on, and sometimes they dishonestly denied ever having received mental health treatment. They avoided contact with others, social situations, job seeking, or even psychiatric treatment in order to avoid risk of disclosure of mental illnesses. In addition to those who wrote or reported such inclinations without prompting, seventeen of our one hundred interviewees explicitly said, in response to our strategy question, that they utilized avoidance, withdrawal, or concealment as coping strategies. Interviewees offered these comments about nondisclosure: "The primary strategy for me is not disclosing." "Another way of dealing with the stigma, I guess, has just been to not bring it up." "Most of the time I don't say anything about my problem to people." One consumer managed to protect himself from stigma by confining his interactions to the internet; his strategy, he said, was "just stay home. If I want to talk to someone, talk to someone on the internet where they can't see you. They don't know nothing about you."

Such comments are consistent with previous research that has identified concealment as a common response to stigma. A questionnaire study of members of Freedom From Fear, a consumer support group in Staten Island, New York, found that 89 percent of the 245 members responding said that they had withheld information on their disorders in response to stigma; 9 percent reported that not even close family members knew of their disorders.[3] Secrecy and withdrawal were two of three major coping strategies identified by Bruce Link and his colleagues in their 1991 interviews with consumers from the Washington Heights section of New York City.[4] Unfortunately, as noted previously, subsequent research by Link also raised questions about the effectiveness of these avoidance strategies. Findings suggested, in fact, that secrecy and withdrawal might have harmful, rather than beneficial effects, leading to greater demoralization and less success finding employment.[5]

When Nancy Herman interviewed 146 persons recently discharged from Canadian hospitals, she reported that nearly 80 percent of those individuals engaged in some form of information control to manage stigma. However, the strategies she identified were less extreme versions of the concealment strategies identified by others. These included what she called "selective concealment" (avoiding disclosure in specific circumstances where the possibility of stigma and discrimination were judged high), "therapeutic disclosure" (disclosure to a trusted few for catharsis and support), and "preventive disclosure" (revelation of psychiatric status early in a relationship and framed in a manner intended to reduce negative reactions).[6]

These limited (and perhaps more successful) versions of concealment were described by many of our interviewees.[7] For instance, some individuals chose to disclose only to a limited number of people; they selected those people carefully as those whom they believed would be more likely to understand and/or to provide support rather than ridicule. One consumer described this as "selecting certain key individuals that play a role in my life to tell them exactly what really happened." Another explained, "I don't talk with a lot of people about it unless I really know them well." Often the people to whom consumers chose to disclose were relatives or other mental health consumers. "I can talk to my husband about it," explained one consumer. "Confiding in him has been a strategy."

Often timing figured as part of this selective disclosure strategy. "I try to let people get to know me when I'm not sick," explained one woman, "and then come back and talk about whatever questions they might have." Another said: "I have learned to make friends with people but not to immediately give them that kind of background because it really does color the way they see you, and some people would not even pursue a friendship like that. . . . I just take the time to develop the friendship and for them to get to know me and like me for who I am, and they seem to be a little more open and a little more accepting that I have an illness." Another aspect of selective disclosure involved *how* consumers talked about their illnesses; they tried to provide information that might lessen fears and misconceptions. "If I tell someone, I'll explain it to them, what it is, and try to explain what it's about," noted one man.

Interviewees also reported using a strategy that is probably a version of what Herman dubbed "preventive disclosure." Consumers sometimes used a sort of first-strike, let's-get-it-over-with approach in which they told others immediately about their mental illness to generate understanding and sympathy, as well as to avoid disappointments later on. "Telling people right off. Just telling people right off in not a scary way," explained one interviewee. "So I just tell them that I suffer from major depression, and I have to be very, very careful with stress." "I've just been very honest with people," said another interviewee utilizing this approach, "and you either like me as I am or the hell with you." Another put it this way: "Those who accept me as I am, we remain friends. Those who can't, 'bye' because I'm not going to pursue relationships based on performing to their standards."

Seeking support from others was also a strategy described by many interviewees. Sixteen of those interviewed indicated that they had found involvement with other mental health consumers to be helpful to them. They sought out others with mental illnesses for support and understanding. "Part of [my strategy] is trying to find people that support me and putting myself in situations where I'm accepted," explained one consumer. Another noted, "Seeing someone who's gone through a lot of what you have and has had to deal with a lot of the same things, including stigma and discrimination, on the job or wherever is just really, really helpful." Consumers often found such contacts through regular attendance at consumer support groups. "People need these small groups, like my Schizophrenics Anonymous group," said one woman. "It's incredibly helpful." Consumers valued these groups because they felt that other consumers would understand better what they were experiencing and would be less judgmental and more supportive than nonconsumers. In addition, consumer support groups, which many interviewees said they attended, provided them the opportunity to help others like themselves, an experience that is both empowering and self-esteem enhancing. Said one man: "It does help to have other people that are in your boat say what's bothering them and you hear what other people have problems with and you try to help them with their problems."

Consumers sought and received emotional support from sources other than fellow consumers, however. As might be expected, they cited the comfort and support received from family, friends, and therapists. In addition, despite some unfavorable experiences people reported from churches, several people emphasized that their religions and their church involvements were important in helping them to cope: "I have very strong spiritual faith," said one interviewee, adding that "God has not put us in situations that we cannot endure." "I also have a strong spiritual base," explained another, "so I do a lot of praying." A third indicated that "I have become a Christian since I started having the problem and that has helped me."

Another strategy that consumers described was self-education about mental illness. Consumers sought to learn as much as they could about their mental illnesses so that they would be less susceptible to the misconceptions that abound about mental disorder. "I'm a member of a support group for people with mental illness and we talk about it," said one interviewee. "And I educate myself about the illness and read and try to gather information to keep myself up-to-date." Another explained: "I guess [my strategy has been] just learning as much as I can. . . . I think the more knowledge that I have, the more my knowledge base has grown, the easier that it's been." "I've tried to educate myself," said still another. "I've done a lot of reading in the past year about depression. . . . I joined NAMI. I attended the meetings and listened to other people, [and it's helped] knowing that it's not just me that has problems." A fourth stated similarly that an important part of her strategy was "becoming as educated as I can. . . . I've worked very hard at learning as much and reading as much as I can."

Sometimes, the efforts at self-education were part of a larger effort at illness management and overall self-improvement. Consumers conveyed that attending to their own health was important to dealing with stigma; successfully managing one's illness and maintaining their self-confidence and self-esteem through such success made it less likely that they would be overwhelmed by stigma. Thus, many consumers responded to our questions about personal strategies for dealing with stigma by citing the many things they did to maintain good mental health. This included adherence to therapy regimens, attending support group meetings, engaging in esteem-enhancing activities, and so on. Typical comments from consumers included: "Continuing to stay in therapy. To continue to work with my therapist. New drugs. To attend the monthly meetings of the local chapter of NAMI. And to volunteer." "I think one of the most important [strategies] is to get something constructive to do. If you're no more than going to volunteer two or three hours a week at a church or school or something, [it will] make for better understanding with yourself and build self-esteem." "I've talked to therapy people. I've gone to all my doctor's appointments. I've talked to my case management people." "I go to the mood challenged group. I see my therapist when I feel I need to. I try to keep on my medicine. I keep myself as busy as possible. I go to singles meetings. I go visit my friends and I just try to keep busy. And I walk and go dancing." "Just having a job and being able to go there every day and doing a good job. . . . I can't tell you how important it's been. It's really helped not only to be myself and open with [others] but to have a job and make money and improve self-esteem and self-confidence and the whole thing."

Two things are particularly noteworthy in this type of remark from consumers. First, it is apparent that consumers were not only active in attempting to cope with illness and stigma, but that they were working hard and were strongly committed to improving their lives through their own efforts. Second, they emphasized the very activities that are often denied consumers—jobs and volunteer positions—as important contributors to self-esteem. These activities can help to maintain a sense of worth that prevents consumers from succumbing to the public attitudes and media messages that suggest they are undeserving of empathy and respect. Yet, as shown in previous chapters, consumers often find themselves excluded from just such activities or they do not pursue them because of discouragement and fears of rejection. Denial of such opportunities, then, presents barriers to recovery from both stigma and mental illness.

A few consumers mentioned miscellaneous other growth and spirit-enhancing strategies. For instance, several indicated that they had found art and writing as useful means to express their feelings, maintain their stability, and allow them a healthy sense of accomplishment. "I do artwork," confided a man with schizoaffective and anxiety disorders. "That's the thing that kind of keeps me feeling good about myself." One consumer mailed an article she had written for a mental health magazine. Another sent an entire published book recounting his mistreatment as a mental health consumer.

Sometimes these self-enhancement efforts involved what psychologists would consider cognitive strategies. Consumers reconceptualized the things that happened to them in less negative terms, reassured themselves of their worth, and tried, in those ways, to minimize the internalizing of stigma. "I do a lot of self-talk," said one woman. "And try not to let [what people say] affect me personally." "Rationalization," declared another. "I rely on the fact that I know I'm just as good as anybody else, in the eyes of God, in the eyes of myself." A third explained: "I think that's a very important thing for everyone to realize, that whether or not I was a manic-depressive or still am, the way I was treated was totally uncalled for." One consumer indicated that she had found it useful to record such self-assuring thoughts: "I do things like affirmative statements that I write in my journal every night. . . . I do lots and lots of things to reinforce that I am a human being, that I have value." Consumers also found it helpful to remind themselves that mental illness was only one part of themselves. "To let myself know that it just exists," stated one woman, "that it's just one more factor that I need to deal with." "First and foremost," said another, "accept the fact that you have the illness. And then from that point I would say move on to the point of just thinking that and knowing that this is only one segment of your life."

Reframing people's hurtful remarks in terms of their lack of knowledge rather than consumer inadequacy was another specific cognitive strategy mentioned. "I realize that a lot of the things that people do and say is ignorance," was how one consumer put it. Another explained: "It used to hurt me that I thought I had people close to me that didn't care about me. And then I realized they're the way they are because they got problems. And that, if they come up with some crap, I just don't have to buy it." Part of this self-instructional strategy was also reminding themselves not to become upset by the stigma they encountered. "I just try to let things go, what people say," explained one interviewee. "Because people are going to talk about you regardless of how you are. So I just try to take it easy and not to worry about what people say about me."

The most commonly reported strategy for dealing with stigma was some form of advocacy, claimed by forty-four of our one hundred interviewees.[8] As discussed in the previous chapter, stigma experiences—and the hurt and anger they engendered—motivated many consumers to work for change as a way of fighting back. This emotion-fueled determination combined with a rational recognition that reducing stigma would be in the best interests of themselves and other consumers who faced such stigma. In addition, comments indicated that some consumers felt an obligation, by virtue of their having greater understanding of mental illness, stigma, and their effects, to contribute to changing attitudes. Finally, consumers engaged in advocacy and public education activities because such activities reduced their feelings of impotence and victimization; it felt good to them and greatly bolstered their self-image to be someone who could help others rather than simply to be someone who needed help.

Consumers became involved in organized activities designed to combat public misunderstanding of mental illness. "I'm active in NAMI," noted one consumer. "When they come out with new posters and stuff, I make sure that the hospital has a supply. They come out with buttons, I wear those and explain what they mean." "I was involved in an organization that did educational programs," recounted another activist. "I felt like, the more people I reach, then maybe it might not make it easier for me, but it's going to make it easier for someone. Because someday, when somebody has to tell or decides to tell someone else that they have this disease, they're going to say, 'Oh, yeah. When I was in high school, these people came in and talked to us, and, yeah, I know about this.'"

They also undertook their own educational and antistigma actions. "I started a supportive and educational group for people with mental illness and their families," said one woman. "We try to go out and do things in the community just because I feel that, once we have contact with them and they see what we're really like, they would be more accepting." Another woman reported that "we started the Stamp Out Stigma program here. . . . We do a lot of graduate schools, schools of nursing, police departments, fire departments. . . . And we try to help the police and fire departments find humane ways of taking people to the hospital. . . . We all feel very rewarded with the work we do. Even, we just feel it's reducing, to some degree, some barriers." Still another used computer technology to accomplish the goal of educating others. "I got my Web page," she reported, "and I try to provide information or links to information to educate people about mental illness."

In contrast to many consumers' strategy of concealment, many other consumers spoke up when they encountered ignorance or misstatements about mental illness. They did this to combat future stigma by educating others and encouraging more accepting behavior, but also they found the experience generally empowering. It felt good to speak up rather then suffer silently. It gave them a sense of satisfaction that they were not too intimidated to speak. And, perhaps more important, it helped them to feel good about themselves as contributors to a larger and worthy cause; they could see themselves as helping not only themselves but other consumers. Many indicated that they wrote letters to government officials urging support of improved mental health legislation and/or to media personnel and advertisers objecting to negative stereotypes witnessed. One consumer summarized what he did: "By writing letters to congressmen and senators and politicians, I try to counterbalance the negative thinking, the stigma about mental illness. I do what I can to make people change their minds." Others were even bolder and spoke directly to stigmatizers. One woman, for instance, characterized herself as "a squeaky wheel in a nice way," adding, "I'm just very confrontive . . . in a nice way, not in an angry way." "I've gotten to a point," stated another woman, "where I will speak out and tell people that what they're saying is really ignorant and they don't really understand." Said a third: "I just will correct people. . . . I'll just say something must have really happened to that person for them to be that way. Don't judge them. Just say things that will help."

Consumers indicated also that they felt that their general willingness to talk publicly about their illnesses was helpful in allowing them to feel less stigmatized. When they could acknowledge their illness without shame or embarrassment, it was liberating. "I think definitely coming out of the closet is one of the most freeing things a person can do," declared one consumer. "I do try to educate people I'm around," said another. "Cause it reinforces that I can educate. I can do something. I don't have to be ashamed of what I deal with." Moreover, consumers felt that sharing their knowledge and perspectives as mental health consumers was a unique and valuable contribution to the education of others and thus enhanced their own feelings of worth as providers of such useful information. Take, for example, the incident described by a woman with bipolar disorder: "They had an American Psychiatric Association meeting [I attended]. And in the evening I was seated . . . next to a gentleman from Scotland. . . . He asked me why I was there. Was I a doctor? I said, 'No. I'm the person they treat. I have a mental illness.' And here's this foreigner from Scotland that doesn't know what mental illness is, but, by the time I was finished, he had an education. So I feel like as if it has empowered me. It helps me erase the stigma for other people."

In addition, consumers were aware that their visibility as reasonably well-functioning consumers helped to contradict some negative expectations others have about mental illness. The good feelings generated by serving as educational role models, along with the acceptance and respect that often followed from their efforts, helped to counteract the negative effects of stigma. "By letting them know [I am a consumer], now they can see that everybody that's had problems isn't running around with an axe in their hand," explained one man with schizoaffective disorder. "I think I'm a fairly rational person, and, if I can portray that to them, they might have a better insight of people that's had [mental illness]. . . . Hopefully, I'm helping others. If you're accepted by people that don't know it and then you tell them, . . . then they're going to say, 'Well, gee, I never realized that people that have problems can be this rational, sensible, not flying off the handle.' Then it makes everybody look better. It makes them more willing to accept the next person." "I try in my personal life to be a kind of crusader," said another, "and tell my friends, 'Hey, this is what I've gone through.' I go around and try to be an example of 'Hey, I can do this and this and this, and I'm one of the people that you think would not be able to do that.'" A third suggested that "part of the purpose of my life right now I feel is to just be the best men-tally ill person that I can be so that people will see me and then know me and then find out that I'm manic-depressive and then go 'Oh, Wow! Maybe not all mentally ill people are completely out of it.'"

Stigma is a problem not just for individuals with psychiatric dis-orders: it is a challenge for the entire mental health field and for society as a whole. How to reduce stigma for the future is therefore an important question. And, in searching or planning for strategies to reduce stigma and discrimination against those with mental ill-nesses, it would be wise to include the wisdom of those who have faced such stigma and discrimination. Accordingly, our interview also included a question about consumer suggestions for how to deal with the problem. Specifically, we asked each of our one hundred interviewees, "What do you think needs to be done to reduce the stigma of mental illness?"

Only the few consumers who were without suggestions expressed an unchecked pessimism that anything could be accomplished. "I don't think anything can be done," said one man. "People have al-ready made up their minds." "I see it as kind of hopeless," said an-other. "It's been there so long, and it's still there, and I think it probably always will be." A couple offered some angry (but not necessarily ineffective) solutions: "I think some of the politicians should be sent to mandatory confinement or involuntary confinement." "I think everybody needs to have [mental illness] once so they'll understand it. I think that's the only way. It seems folks do not really understand it unless it happens to them."

By far, the most common strategy recommended, by two-thirds of our interviewees, was education about mental illness. Consumers believed that, if people understood more about mental disorders and about what it was like to have a psychiatric disorder, then they would not be so quick to make disparaging remarks or show such reluc-tance to employ or befriend them. "Educate people," said one woman. "I think it's mostly through ignorance and fear that, like any type of prejudice, if you can present things positively, disseminate informa-tion in a positive manner, that people will accept it and be less afraid." Several consumers also voiced the view that such education should ideally begin in childhood. As one consumer put it: "Education needs to start with people when they are children. [Teach] that there are people with different types of disabilities and just because they've got a disability doesn't mean that they don't have the right to be treated the same. Respect needs to be taught."

A number of consumers suggested that public education was needed on a grand scale—efforts involving corporate commitment and generous funding. "I don't think it's unreasonable to suggest," opined one man, "that the stigma issue should be near the top of the list for educators. . . . I think until we get to the point where we're willing to spend that kind of money. . . . The stigma issue is so important that I think a large corporate effort is required." "Enormous public education," another suggested similarly, "through high-profile programs [like] campaigns that have required literally millions of dollars. Something on that level would be needed for mental illness."[9]

Other consumers felt that such education required a more specific target than a campaign aimed at the general public. Many interviewees suggested that education should be directed at specific groups that they saw as either particularly likely to be involved with consumers or particularly egregious in their stigmatizing actions. Mental health professionals were one such group. "It should start with the doctors," asserted one woman, "it should start in medical school. Say 'Hey, you people need to learn how to treat people like people.' Reeducate the doctors that have been psychiatrists for long times."[10] Another group mentioned repeatedly as a target for education was that of media professionals. "I think that as soon as we start educating people like the people who are doing our national news and the people who are reporting the news," explained an interviewee, "that the plight of people with mental illness will be somewhat less of a burden."[11] Other groups mentioned included churches, law enforcement agents, politicians, and educators.

The media was mentioned not only as a place where education was needed but also as a means for providing more public education and a way to reach large numbers of people with corrective information about mental illness. One person even suggested that "the only thing we pay attention to, I think, in popular culture is television and that sort of thing. I think it has far more effect on the standard person, the average person."

"People have to get to these talk shows," was one typical recommendation. "That's a big forum for people every day, like 'Talk Back Live' and 'Oprah Winfrey.' And get some discussions on some kind of shows because it seems that they attract a very wide audience. Television and radio would probably be good." "More articles, and more, like *Oprah*, more talk shows," suggested another consumer.[12] "I think people need to be educated," said a fourth, echoing the common theme. "There needs to be a few programs about it so people will understand. But it's the type of thing where there's very few programs that are actually on television. . . . If they'd do a documentary or something."[13] Other consumers were even more ambitious: "If we could get a commercial on the Superbowl, they could be touching billions of people."[14] "I think the president needs to talk about it. I think the governor and the president and the mayors, they ought to talk about it on the news."[15]

A related strategy was the use of celebrity spokespersons. Some consumers felt that the willingness of people with stature and wide public recognition who also have mental disorders to disclose and talk about their mental illnesses would be particularly helpful. Such individuals, it was believed, would attract more attention to messages about mental illness and thus enhance public education efforts. In addition, consumers expected that knowledge that well-known and admired celebrities had mental illnesses might increase overall acceptance of those illnesses. "If there were things like if Kay Jamison's book or Martha Manning's book were made into movies or television movies, I think that would help," offered one interviewee.[16] "The kind of thing that really talks to people, that kinda gets them more. . . . [like] those ads they had with Winston Churchill and Abraham Lincoln, I think those were good."[17] "More needs to be spoken," said another. "People like Jamison need to go on, go and talk. Mike Wallace . . . and Naomi Judd and Art Buchwald."[18] Still another observed: "As people of importance share that they have these problems, that draws attention. I know Margot Kidder recently came out. . . . And I know Patty Duke."[19]

Many consumers expressed the belief that successful treatment of mental illness was the key to stigma reduction. Greater accessibility of treatment, improved methods for reducing symptoms and behaviors that frighten the public, adequate housing and employment to free people with mental illnesses from homelessness and dependency were seen as keys to changing the public image of mental illness. It is easier to be accepted, consumers reasoned, if one is functioning well. As one interviewee noted: "If somebody's walking around sick as a dog, they're going to scare people, and miss work, and mess up. So, actually, just putting some of this energy into getting the treatment across to people that need it." "I think [stigma] will change when they find a cure," explained another. "Because one thing we know is that people don't want to be like us. This is something nobody wants, kind of like leprosy. So if you can't do anything about it, it's more frightening than something you can do something with. So I think when there's something that can be done about it that's definitive and it works every time for everybody, it will be better." "I think if people were given proper care that they would not act in a way to appear crazy," said a third in response to our strategy question.

Thus, consumer recommendations for strategies to reduce stigma included many calls for increased resources to permit people with mental illness to recover. "Starting and sustaining projects that help people with mental illnesses cope better," recommended one man. "Successful projects . . . and funding for programs that work." Consumers also recognized that money for research that might lead to better understanding and treatment of mental illness was needed. For instance, one consumer asserted: "More money needs to be spent on research on mental illness. There should be a campaign to raise that money just like we raise money for cancer. We should have an organization like the American Cancer Society or Heart Association or something like that for mental illness to raise money for research."[20] Legal actions—to require insurance parity and to permit legal redress of maltreatment—were also recommended.[21]

Moreover, consumers suggested a strategy to confront and challenge stigmatizers; their goal was not only to communicate disapproval but also to educate those demonstrating ignorance and misunderstanding. Some wanted advocacy organizations to lead the way in confronting stigmatizers: "It's almost as if there needs to be an office associated with some, either the American Psychiatric Association or the American Medical Association, someone whose job it is to search down every piece of information and write a correction."[22] Others felt that consumers themselves should do the challenging: "Consumers need to get out and be more active and respond when they see that there's some kind of negative stereotype that's being conveyed," said a typical consumer. "I think responding back and educating," said another. "Not responding back with smart remarks but trying to educate people." In fact, many consumers did respond back, as they described in their descriptions of their personal coping strategies. They wrote letters to editors, advertisers, and TV stations about offending depictions of mental illness. They talked about how they "correct people" and how they have been "able to express to people my anger when I see [stigma]." One noted that "if I hear someone say something that is inaccurate about mental illness, I will be happy to inform them that is not exactly the way it is." A few reported that they had taken legal actions by calling upon Americans with Disabilities Act (ADA) and Equal Employment Opportunity Commission (EEOC) protections to correct perceived discrimination.[23]

The tenacity displayed by some consumers in their work to redress stigma is shown in the efforts reported by the consumer whose experience with a Young Leaders program was described in chapter 6. She was troubled, readers may recall, by a volunteer application form that specified that anyone being treated for mental illness would not be admitted as a volunteer for the program because "experience has shown that this can be harmful to these youth and adults." Her determined response included the following:

> After much thought, I decided that it was best to simply not answer the questions on this part of the application form. I wrote a lengthy paragraph explaining that, as a member of a number of mental health organizations, I found this section discriminatory and in violation of the Americans with Disabilities Act. No one said anything about the application, either the missing information or the statement. I went to camp. Everything went great. In December of 1995, our school district was again invited to participate. . . . I received all the information I needed to once again organize my school district's involvement. Absolute anger cannot

begin to describe my feelings on again seeing the same discriminatory statement in the volunteer staff member application form.
Since I had to call the program organizer . . . to discuss some
timelines, I thought I'd also bring up this section of the application. [She] greeted me cordially and immediately asked if I would
once again serve on the staff. I told her I really couldn't because
of [her organization's] statement about mental illness. She assured me that I could of course attend because she knew that I
was 'OK.' She had 'heard' my points about how this statement
was discriminatory . . . but, by the time I hung up, it was clear
that she intended to leave the application as it was. . . . Well,
I've had it. The application is downright insulting. This year I
intend to revise the application myself, eliminating that section
entirely.

Confrontation and challenge, however, require considerable
confidence and courage, and perhaps a thick skin. Thus, many consumers, while identifying consumer actions as very important in com-
bating stigma, suggested less demanding contributions. Many
recommended (in line with the personal strategies described earlier)
that simple increased visibility of people with mental illness—not
just celebrities, but ordinary people with psychiatric disorders—could
be substantially helpful in reducing stigma in several ways. Consumers suggested that they themselves could be instructive in educating
others about mental illness: their first-hand knowledge of psychiatric disorder enabled them to best describe the experience of mental
illness. Being available as educators would also allow others to see
persons with mental illness in different roles and perhaps be less
threatened by and more accepting of mental illness as a result. "I
would suggest things like a Speakers' Bureau," said an interviewee,
"where people who have mental illnesses go into classrooms or go to
organizations and talk about the illness. . . . I think we need to go out
there ourselves and say, 'Look, meet me, here I am; I'm an okay person.'"[24] "I think it would be good if there was more literature available to people," began another interviewee. "And what might be even
better is the availability for people who really wanted to know to

have someone to talk to who has that illness and can explain it to them."[25]

Consumers expressed the belief that more consumers, particularly those in "normal" settings who have been relatively successful in managing their illnesses, need to be visible to challenge others' misconceptions about mental illness. "One of the important things is for consumers to . . . go out in the world and show the world what they can do," explained one woman. "And I think it's important that people that have mental illnesses that are functioning in society at high levels speak up about their illness. . . . If you're out there working with people, then they see you first-hand . . . and you're counteracting the stigma that you're worthless because you have a mental illness." Said another: "The more people speak out about it, the more people may realize that they already know mentally ill people who just haven't been willing to take the risk of sharing that." Another consumer said similarly: "I think more people that have mental illness have to admit it. I see many people be affected by mental illness, get on appropriate medication, recover from the symptoms, and never again admit or say that they have a mental illness. So those around them just see them as a normal person, and since they will never say otherwise, no one ever knows that people can have a mental illness, get the proper medicine, and then be 'normal.'"

This strategy of consumer disclosure, of course, may be more easily prescribed than carried out. The widespread experiences of stigma and discrimination reveal clearly that "telling is risky business," as one of our survey participants observed.[26] Those who have achieved status and comfort have much to lose by revealing their stigmatized psychiatric condition. Those who are struggling to maintain stability may be unable to risk the possible additional burdens of negative attitudes and discrimination. Indeed, three-quarters of our survey participants indicated that they at least sometimes concealed their disorders from others. Nevertheless, even those who were neither able to overcome their fears nor willing to disclose in certain situations seemed to disagree that consumer visibility and openness about psychiatric disorder—although difficult to manage—could be a valuable strategy for reducing stigma.[27]

A few consumers expressed an even stronger view: disclosure was an obligation for consumers concerned about stigma. "I realize," said one person, "that I have to tell people or I'm adding to the stigma. If I can't admit it, how can I expect other people to understand?" "If people don't speak out," said another simply, "then it continues." A third asserted: "If I don't start trying to speak out, then I'm part of the problem as opposed to part of the solution." Still another expressed the opinion that "in a way, everyone needs to be a poster child because we're not someone you don't know. Not everyone's ready to disclose . . . but if more people did, there wouldn't be the idea that it's a secret and it's shameful." There was, in fact, repeated recognition that disclosure is essential to challenge the view of mental illness as something shameful and best hidden: "As long as the people themselves, the people with mental illness and the families who have a loved one with mental illness, as long as they consider it to be a stigma, they're continuing to promote stigma by their silence."

The voices of consumers tell us that they have many ideas and have taken many actions to deal with stigma, in terms of both their own personal day-to-day coping and their efforts to reduce stigma within society. Consumers reported a number of ways they actively sought to deal with the stigma and the corresponding discrimination. Their strategies included self-protective concealment of their consumer status, selective disclosure to only those people (such as other consumers) judged likely to be more understanding and less judgmental, and preventive disclosure in which they let others know right away about their illness so that they could find out quickly which relationships to pursue. Their personal coping efforts included also general health and mental health maintenance, self-expression activities such as writing and painting, and cognitive strategies such as positive self-instruction and reminders that the ignorance of others should not sway their self-assessments. Many consumers reported involvement in advocacy to be for them an esteem-enhancing activity that helped to counteract the feelings generated by the negative attitudes and treatment they encountered. Consumers felt empowered by such activities: they were now able to take action to challenge or correct the stigmatizing situations they faced, to establish and reassure themselves of their competence, and to help not only themselves but also others.

Consumers offered many thoughtful suggestions about challenging and reducing stigma in the future. They saw education about mental illness as a key element, particularly educating people in the mental health field and young people whose views are still in the formative stages. Consumers also recommended challenging and confronting stigma and discrimination when they occur—through legislation, legal actions, and personal response. Involving consumers in such education and challenge, moreover, was seen as important, if not obligatory. In particular, people felt that successful consumers— of both celebrity and noncelebrity status—needed to be visible and outspoken to provide direct, living disconfirmation of the public's negative views and expectations about those with mental illnesses.

10

Consumer

Messages about

Mental Illness

In conducting a nationwide survey of consumers we had two main goals. We tried to gain a better understanding of the extent to which stigma and discrimination continue to be part of the lives of people with mental illnesses. And we offered consumers a rare opportunity to speak and be heard concerning their experiences and their ideas about stigma. In the fulfillment of both of these goals, then, we ended each interview by explicitly asking each consumer to tell us what he/she would want us and others to know about mental illness. Specifically, we asked each interviewee the following question at the end of his/her interview: "If there was one message you could give people about mental illness, one request you could make to them, what would it be?" For those who truly wish to be open to consumer input and to know what consumers think is important to understand about mental illnesses—not just what mental health professionals or academics or family members think, but what those who have struggled firsthand with mental illness believe—interviewee responses to this question may be among the most important results of our project.

Consumers primarily asked others to be more caring and supportive toward them. As the experiences of rejection and exclusion recounted in previous chapters suggest, many consumers found empathy lacking. Recognizing that such support is needed by them, especially at times during their illnesses when they felt overwhelmed and discouraged, consumers called upon others to "be kind, loving, understanding, sensitive." Another consumer's chosen message was that "mentally ill people need your support and encouragement just as any people need with any illness." "Because we are weak," said a third, "when we suffer a lot of psychic pain, it's difficult for us to raise our voices to ask you to be kind to us because we are very fragile. And we need your support." "Try to be more compassionate," suggested a fourth, while still another asked others "to be a little bit more understanding and patient with people that are different."

Consumers also seemed to feel that nonconsumers often did not appreciate the sheer difficulty of living with a mental illness and called for empathic appreciation of their lives and struggles with both mental illness and its stigma. One person's message, for instance, was: "The suffering of mental illness is just incredible. . . . The suffering. I can't emphasize that enough because I think a physical affliction would never have been as painful as mental illness. Because of the stigma, because of people turning their backs and walking away. It's like somebody stepping over a dead body. If you were dying on the street, literally dying, and people just kinda blasé and stepped over you . . . how would you feel?" Another person urged others to "think about if it was you in that situation. How would you feel if you were being treated the way you are treating people in that situation. . . . Try placing yourself in the situation of a person with mental illness and how they are treated—about being shunned and put down as if they don't belong in society. Just put yourself in that place for one hour or one day and see how it feels." A third said that what she wanted to tell others was: "Try to understand the pain that's involved with [mental illness] and the support that people need during depressive episodes or hospitalizations. I think I want people to know the struggle of day-to-day life and keeping your head above the water." A fourth simply wanted people to know "that it is very, very painful—emotionally, spiritually, socially."

Several consumers urged empathy by offering messages that emphasized that mental illness could happen to anyone. As one interviewee explained: "These illnesses can hit anybody any time. And there but for the grace of God go I as far as what patients are. I think people need to know that these illnesses can hit anybody any time. And just because they think they're doing all that great and grand doesn't mean a week from now they won't be suffering." Another said similarly: "Anybody can have mental health problems, and anyone could be in the same boat." "Please try to develop some patience," advised a third interviewee, "because it could be you tomorrow." Still another consumer's warning was even more direct and personal: "Don't laugh. It may happen to you." Consumers also pointed out that mental illness can—and often does—affect one's loved ones: "A consumer could be your brother, could be your sister, could be your mother, your father, could be yourself. And you need to be aware of that." "You never know it might happen to you or someone in your family. Because it doesn't pick on the poor, the rich, black, white, or whatever. . . . It would be wise to try and understand it better."

Consumers' messages suggested that they also wanted people to understand specific things about mental illness. Some, for example, wanted others to understand that not all people with mental illnesses are violent or out of control: "There's a vast difference between people with mental illness and those people who are criminally insane. . . . I don't want people to equate people with mental illness and people in jail." "Taking an antidepressant doesn't mean somebody's out of control or about to freak out or needs to be hospitalized." "It's a very lonely illness and I think that it's lonely because people are afraid of us, and that's the other thing I want to tell people is, there's nothing to be afraid of, there's nothing to be afraid of from us." "The vast majority of people with mental illness are not dangerous."

Consumers expressed their secondary desire for others to understand that mental illness is a "real" disease, not just a lapse in motivation, a developmental phase, or a ploy to gain sympathy. This very important message from consumers was not surprising when considering the reports in previous chapters of consumers' painful illnesses being discounted by others. They sought to have others recognize mental illness as real: sometimes they asserted that mental illnesses are genetic or biological in nature; sometimes they compared their illnesses to other medical conditions and identified the brain as the afflicted organ. "Mental illness is a disease like any other disease, and it should be portrayed as such," was a typical statement. "It's an illness just like anything else," said another interviewee. "It just affects a different part of the body." A third said he wanted people to know "that it's a brain chemical disorder. That it's a disease like any other."

Biological causation was stressed also to convey that mental illness is a "no-fault" disease, produced by neither the individual's lack of will or character or faith nor the actions of parents or spouses: "Understand that it is a physical illness; it's not a choice. It's not a weakness, a moral choice. It's just like any other illness." "Mental illness is a chemical imbalance and brain disorder. It's not something in the imagination or something because we're lazy or stupid." "Try to understand that it's not a question of willpower, that it can't be mind over matter." "If it were a matter of thinking the right things and feeling the right way, I would be well. But it's not." "Mental illness is no one's fault. It's inherited. It's biological. It's genetic, just as the color of your hair and the color of your eyes and your body shape. . . . You don't do anything to bring it on yourself. Your wife doesn't bring it on, your spouse doesn't bring it on. There's no blame; no blame has to be placed on anybody. It's a no-fault disease. It's a no-blame disease any more than you'd blame somebody for getting cancer or diabetes." Consumers also asserted the biological nature of the illness to convey that psychiatric treatment was a necessity, not an indulgence. "Mental illness is a brain disease. It requires psychiatric care and medication. And it's for real."

Consumers were also concerned that others often do not get beyond their stereotyped images of mental illness and that people tend to respond to consumers based on preconceived notions (and/or media images) of what a person with mental illness will be like. One of the more common requests voiced by consumers, then, was a call for reduced judgment or prejudgment of consumers based upon either their diagnostic label or stereotypes of mental illness: "You shouldn't judge on the basis of your own stereotype." "Be willing to be awakened to what is really happening with people with mental illness. Don't just blindly submit yourself to the stereotypical mode that's trying to be enforced upon us." "Just try to understand it. Don't take the preconceived notions. Don't take these portrayals of people as gospel." "Just because someone has a label, don't think they're going to act in a certain way." "Until you've walked in their shoes, don't justify or rationalize writing them off as human beings."

The theme of "walking in our shoes," in fact, was used repeatedly by consumers in their requests for others to neither judge nor reject them: "Don't judge me until you've walked a mile in my shoes. Instead of just passing judgment on me by looking at me and saying, 'Well, she's mentally ill; she's just not right in her mind' or something like that, I think they ought to stop and think about it before they speak. Words are hurtful. And actions are even worse. But I think that's what I would tell them is just stop and don't judge people." "Don't criticize me unless you've walked in my shoes for a couple of years. Unless you've walked in my shoes, you don't know what I've been through."

Still other consumers asked not just for compassion, understanding, and nonjudgmental viewing, but they also requested active efforts from the public to learn about mental illness and to engage in or support work that would benefit those with psychiatric disorders. "Please study, get educated," was what one person requested. "Learn what mental illness is. Once they learn, then it's a different story. . . . And if you know a person with mental illness, learn about it, get educated about it." Learning from consumers themselves was particularly recommended: "Read any literature you can by consumers," urged one interviewee. "And attend as many consumer conferences as you can just to educate yourself. . . . Get involved with consumers." Another asked that others "listen to people and really try to understand what the other person's going through."

Consumers suggested also that, beyond taking steps to learn more about mental illnesses, the public could do a better job of supporting consumer efforts to recover. They suggested, for example, that others could help them advocate for improved care: "Demand better treatment and better services to help [consumers] toward becoming more productive people." Consumers also asked for opportunities to help themselves and to prove themselves to the community. "Give us a chance," said one man. "You give us a chance, we are productive, and, there's so many of us, we can contribute so much to the nation, to the state, to the country, to the city. Just give us a chance." "Consumers are not looking for handouts," noted another, "but consumers are looking for opportunities. They're looking for employment opportunities, looking for advocacy opportunities, looking for housing opportunities."

Probably the most common—and most impassioned—message from consumers involved requests to be valued as human beings and to be accorded the respect and dignity to which all human beings should be entitled: "Try to be understanding and compassionate. Whenever [you] hear that somebody's got a mental illness, don't act like they've died or like they're worthless or they're no good anymore, they're ruined. . . . Esteem them as valuable human beings." "Accept us as human beings just like them. [Treat us] with the same respect they want to be treated with." "People that have mental illnesses are people too and they deserve respect." "Treat us like you would like to be treated. . . . Everyone should be treated equal, whether you have an illness or not. We should all be treated equal." "Treat me just like someone who has kidney [disease] or cancer or any other illness, with dignity and respect." "We are people too. Consumers are people too."

The demand to be valued as individual human beings included also the expressed desire for others to see the complex individuals they really are. Again, many expressed concern that others did not get beyond their psychiatric labels or their dramatic symptoms and viewed them primarily, if not exclusively, in terms of their illnesses.[1] Consumers, for example, expressed a desire for others to consider *who* (the person) rather than *what* (schizophrenic, manic-depressive, etc.) they are. "Don't judge who we are by the fact that we have a mental illness," said one woman. "Don't judge a person by their sickness," urged another. "Judge them by who they are underneath."

Consumers wanted not just minimal respect as members of the same (human) species but also a recognition and appreciation of the traits and experiences and motives they shared with nonconsumers. Consumers emphasized that they are first and foremost *people with disorders*;[2] underneath their illnesses, they have the same fascinating, frustrating, and diverse characteristics as other people: "People with mental illness, at some time, in some place, are just like everybody else. We got the same wishes and hopes and dreams and we have the same feelings. . . . I'm a person, not a disease." "I think people too often define a person by their illness. And, as we know, that's a very limited way of seeing somebody and there's just lots of stereotypes and stigma and discrimination. . . . Because, I mean, we're in so many ways exactly like other people. I mean, we need friends and meaningful work and leisure time and social activities just like everyone else."

Consumers sometimes bolstered their messages about being like others by pointing out that people probably already know someone with a mental illness who is so like themselves that they do not even realize that the person has a mental illness. One interviewee with much to say explained:

> I think [my message] would be that people with mental illness are people first. . . . Mental illness is just part of them. And that you're probably surrounded by people with mental illness, and you don't even know it. . . . You wouldn't even be able to tell walking up to them on the street. We have to lose this image of crazed lunatics and deinstitutionalized homeless people. . . . Just basically that people with mental illness are more or less the same as other people. They just have this disease that makes it very difficult for them to live their lives. . . . [But] people are functional and they're capable . . . they're capable and they're out there and it's not just child molesters and homeless people or killers or something. It's not just ax murderers. It's like the guy in the cubicle next to you . . . or your son's girlfriend . . . or your mother.

"You know somebody with a mental illness," suggested another. "[You] probably already know somebody with it. It's not that alien to [you], and it's not obvious all the time."

Another facet of these repeated messages from consumers about their common humanity was the reminder that their mental illnesses are just one part of them, not the whole (or even the most important) basis for knowing and relating to them. As one interviewee pointed out in her chosen message: "Mental illness is just a piece of a person. A person is composed of so many more pieces than mental illness. I am more than a diagnosis. I am a whole person, and I deserve to be treated like a whole person, just like you deserve to be treated as a whole person."

Finally, consumers communicated that they deserved respect not just because they were human beings and they shared traits with nonconsumers, but also because they had strengths, talents, and other admirable qualities through which they made valuable contributions to society. As one consumer noted: "We're intelligent enough, and we've got internal strength to overcome whatever situation we've got, and we can live a productive life if allowed to." "We're bright and we're sensitive, maybe even more sensitive than the people looking down at us," another pointed out. "And we see a lot even when we're delusional or psychotic or very sick or very depressed." "Rather than condemn [consumers, people] should reach out a hand to them," explained a third. "There's some pretty neat people."

Consumer messages, then, were neither particularly demanding nor particularly difficult to understand. Consumers indicated that they want support and empathy from others. They want appreciation of the hardships they face, and they seek opportunities that will permit them to improve their lives. They desire not to be stereotyped, not to be prejudged on the basis of inaccurate and unfavorable stereotypes of mental illness, and not to be blamed for the symptoms of illnesses they did not choose. They ask that others respond to them on the basis of their personal characteristics rather than their psychiatric labels, and they implore others to recognize that mental illness is only one part of the people they are. Moreover, they make the most fundamental request of all—to be accorded the respect and dignity that is due to all human beings. Not one of these messages seems in the least outrageous or unreasonable. As do consumers, I hope that such messages will be heard and heeded.

11

Cautions and

Limitations

As with any study, limitations must be acknowledged. There are, for example, significant limitations to any generalization of our results that stem from the self-selected nature of our survey and interview respondents. Even though our study of stigma involved the largest single sample of consumers to date, our participants represent only a small fraction of the millions of people with mental illnesses and only a small proportion even of the many thousands of potential respondents to whom the survey was distributed. We do not know whether those who chose to respond and/or agreed to be interviewed were perhaps those who had experienced more stigma and who were, therefore, more motivated to take the time to participate. Similarly, many of our participants were involved in mental health advocacy; because their involvement helped motivate them to contribute to our study, they could be more informed and more vigilant about stigma than those from whom we did not hear. If our participants were indeed more sensitized to stigma by virtue of greater stigma or advocacy experience than the "average" consumer, then our study might be overestimating the extent of stigma and discrimination.

Those in our study may have been better functioning than the hypothetical average consumer. As reported in chapter 3, a high percentage of them were living independently and had completed college or professional school. In addition, the rate of employment was somewhat higher than what has been reported previously among consumers with comparable disorders.[1] It is possible that such individuals may have been better able to escape stigma and discrimination than those who were more disabled by their illnesses and who did not, for that reason, contribute to our study. Thus, one could argue that our study underestimates the degree of stigma and discrimination experienced by the average consumer.

It is also true that the majority of our survey and interview participants came through sources connected with a particular advocacy group—NAMI. Their involvement with this group might, again, indicate greater knowledge and sensitivity to issues of stigma, either as part of their motivation to become involved with NAMI or through NAMI's extensive educational efforts concerning stigma and discrimination. In addition, some messages chosen by consumers echoed the primary messages of NAMI; in particular, they asserted that mental illnesses are biological in nature. "Mental illnesses are brain disorders" is the primary slogan of NAMI's Campaign to End Discrimination, and the choice of this as a message to others may reflect a NAMI indoctrination that other non–NAMI-affiliated consumers might not have selected or even agreed with.

Other ways that the study is not precisely representative of the entire population of consumers were noted earlier. We had more females than males in our sample, particularly among our one hundred interview participants (seventy-one females), and relatively few Hispanic and Asian respondents. We heard from few consumers who were currently hospitalized and even fewer of those among the substantial homeless population. We cannot be sure how greater inclusion of these classes of consumers might have influenced our overall results, although I expect that the public would be even more likely to respond to these populations—males, minorities, hospitalized individuals, and people ill enough to become homeless—with stigma and discrimination than those in our response sample.

Our sample also tends to be middle-aged and older. Given that most had disorders with adolescent or adult onset, this means that most of our respondents would have had many years to accumulate stigma and discrimination experiences. It also means that they would have had many years to learn to cope with both their illnesses and public responses to them. How this may have affected the picture of

stigma that emerged is uncertain. The perceptions and stigma awareness of people during their early struggles with mental illness may
be quite different from those of the more mature individuals who
dominated our sample. Moreover, there may be cohort effects within
the experience of consumers. That is, those who are growing up and
developing mental illness in the 1990s may have a different experience than those who grew up and developed their illnesses in the
1960s, 1970s, or 1980s.

As we observed earlier, the disorders represented in our sample
tend to be the more severe and persistent mental illnesses—schizophrenia, depression, bipolar disorder—and these disorders led to hospitalization episodes for the vast majority of our respondents. Our
results, then, do not tell us about the experiences of those with less
severe psychiatric disorders, disorders that allowed them to continue
to function in their communities without psychiatric hospitalization. One might expect that those individuals with less dramatic and
less disabling symptoms would experience less stigma and discrimination; however, much previous research on stigma demonstrates
little or no distinction about types of mental illness. In fact, it suggests that the public, without distinguishing among types of mental
illness, responds to a psychiatric label of any kind with similar stereotypes and thus similar stigma,[2] and it is a common experience of
clinicians working solely in outpatient settings that even their clients with milder problems, including marriage and family issues, are
reluctant to seek psychiatric treatment and/or to have it known that
they have done so.[3] It would be useful to know the extent to which
such stigma is experienced by these individuals with less severe disorders, but our study does not provide that information. We must be
cautious, then, about generalizing our results to all individuals who
receive a psychiatric diagnosis or mental health treatment.

We must also acknowledge that our study has relied on self-report;
we have not documented directly the experiences conveyed by consumers. As with any self-report, respondents' perceptions of events
may have been colored by their own sensitivities and needs. Their
recollections from experiences undoubtedly reflect only what stood
out for them; they may not capture all the context or circumstances.
Their recall also may differ from that of others involved in the events

reported; for example, their employers may present a completely different scenario. It is even possible that consumer recollections have been shaped by the symptoms of their disorders: that is, people experiencing depression may be able to recall life experiences in only the bleakest terms, or those with paranoid tendencies may be prone to easily detect malevolence and mistreatment where they may be none.

I want to emphasize, however, that recognizing these possibilities does not justify discounting the reports of consumers. The consistency in what consumers report, in fact, certainly suggests that the experiences described are far from fictional products of distorted thinking. Our impression was, furthermore, that these individuals were good reporters—fair and thoughtful. They were not hesitant to say that they had *not* had some of the experiences we asked about, and they were convincing in their descriptions of the experiences they did report. In addition, what we were seeking, after all, was to understand stigma *from the perspective of the consumer*, and that is certainly what they have provided. Despite the limitations of self-report noted, ignoring these reports as merely biased or distorted would be to continue the stigmatizing devaluation of consumer input.

Our study is likewise limited by dealing with only a few aspects of the experience of people with mental illness and thus hardly provides a full understanding of what it means to have a mental illness. We asked only about stigma and discrimination experiences. We did not ask about the direct and indirect effects of the illnesses themselves, knowledge of which that might lead to better empathic understanding. Mental illnesses interfere with social, educational, and occupational growth. They create roller coasters of emotions, frustration and discouragement, fear and pain, even without stigma and discrimination. Our results do not capture that. They also do not tell about the life compromises consumers must make when their illnesses refuse to remain under control: for example, I know a young woman who works as an exotic dancer, taking off her clothes for men in bars because there is always someone willing to hire her for that even if only for a few months between episodes of illness, or the consumers on limited incomes whose "success" in finding housing means a one-room, roach-infested apartment in a crime-ridden neighborhood. Our results, similarly, do not fully address the dilemma created by the current system of medical benefits through which many consumers are encouraged *not* to attempt work because doing so would result in *loss* of needed disability insurance coverage of psychiatric and other medical care. The sometimes remarkable effort expended by consumers to understand and manage their illnesses is likewise not fully revealed in the information we have obtained and presented.

Our study also does not address the sometimes problematic consequences of psychiatric treatment—the controversial practice of involuntary hospitalization, the unpleasant and sometimes dangerous side effects of treatment medications, the inadequacies of many public care facilities, and the poorly coordinated and underfunded system of mental health care. Unlike other studies, such as that of Deborah Reidy, who focused explicitly on the "stigmatizing aspects of mental health programs,"[4] our study encouraged description of stigma and discrimination experiences in the general community. Although participants included experiences with mental health professionals and mental health settings in their responses, we probably did not learn as much about their treatment experiences as we would have if we had asked more explicitly about them.

Finally, we lack an anchor or yardstick against which to measure the degree of stigma reported by our respondents. It is a matter of interpretation, for instance, whether or not the 26 percent of our respondents who reported being often or very often shunned or avoided by others should be considered "a lot." Perhaps, rather than being concerned by that figure, we should be pleased that a larger percentage (38 percent) said they had seldom or never been shunned or avoided by others because of their consumer status. Perhaps we should be pleased that *only* 15 percent of our respondents reported that they had often or very often been turned down for a job when their consumer status was revealed and that *only* 17 percent had been often or very often denied treatment because of insufficient health insurance.

Lacking previous similar studies, we also cannot say whether the extent of stigma experiences is more or less than in the past. It is possible that the number of consumers reporting stigma and discrimination experiences in this study represents *an improvement* over what consumers experienced in the past. Again, it could be that we should be appreciating a positive change rather than focusing on the number of negative experiences that still occur. We cannot know without a comparable basis of comparison from the past.

However, acknowledgment of this limitation, I believe, does not compel us to lessen our concern about the current stigma and discrimination experiences of mental health consumers, as described by the participants in our study. Whether the 26 percent who report being shunned often or very often is an improvement or not, whether they are fewer than the percentage who report being seldom or never shunned, it is still too many. That 26 percent, extrapolated to the larger population of people with mental illnesses, translates to hundreds of thousands, possibly even millions, of people suffering needlessly. Moreover the painful personal experiences described—of being harassed by others, being left isolated and alone, having medical complaints ignored, witnessing disrespect, fear, and ridicule on all sides, having fundamental rights violated, and, in total, being denied the necessary opportunities for a decent quality life—cannot be judged by quantity alone. Even one, much less hundreds or thousands, of such experiences is unacceptable.

The limitations cited, then, call not for disregarding the stigma experiences reported by this sample of consumers but for filling in the gaps with additional studies. Similar surveys of consumers unconnected with NAMI and of consumers with less severe disorders treated in outpatient settings would be helpful, as would samples of consumers who are younger and more culturally diverse. At the same time, it would be good to reach consumers who may be even more stigmatized and disenfranchised—those in hospitals and on the streets. Finally, continued inquiry about the overall life experiences, not just stigma experiences, of consumers is needed to fully appreciate what mental illness means in the lives of our friends, coworkers, neighbors, and loved ones.

12

Resources for

Fighting Stigma

There can be little doubt that mental illness stigma plagues the lives of those with psychiatric disorders, and sometimes consumers and advocates feel overwhelmed by its extent and persistence. However, stigma does not have to be like the weather—something about which everyone complains but no one can do anything. There are many things that people can do, and are in fact doing, to try to reduce stigma and discrimination against people with mental illness. By building on the suggestions made by consumers in previous chapters, I describe some ways those who are interested may help to combat stigma. For both consumers and nonconsumers, I offer a list of ten things we can do to fight stigma.

Ten Things We Can Do to Fight Stigma

1. Go beyond the stereotypes of mental illness. In line with what consumers emphasized in their messages to others, we can avoid prejudging those with mental illnesses on the basis of societal and media stereotypes. We can recognize that a label of mental illness or schizophrenia or manic depressive tells us little about what to expect from the person with that label. Such labels, for example, certainly do *not* tell us that the person is dangerous or incompetent or an unreliable worker. They do *not* tell us about the person's capacity for friendship or creativity or accomplishment. They do *not* tell us

clearly about his or her specific symptoms or potential for recovery. Resisting the negative stereotypes that often cloud our thinking about mental illness is an important step in reducing stigma.

2. Learn more about mental illness. To the extent that we are better informed about mental illness, we are better able to evaluate and resist the inaccurate negative stereotypes of mental illness that are so common. Many organizations provide educational material about mental illnesses, including brochures, fact sheets, and internet postings. Some primary organizations that supply this information are provided in the Resource List later in this chapter. In addition, some books listed below describe various mental illnesses and their treatment; they may be helpful in understanding those disorders.

3. Learn more about stigma and discrimination. The substantial literature on stigma is only touched upon in the brief review earlier in this book. References to some of that literature have been included throughout this book, and I include below recommendations for additional reading for those who wish to understand how stigma has been studied and addressed. Once again, many organizations in the Resource List also provide information concerning stigma and discrimination.

4. Listen to people who have experienced mental illness. People with mental illnesses are in the best position to tell us how mental illness and stigma affect their lives. As consumers did in our survey, they can describe what they find stigmatizing, what they would like us to know about life with mental illness, and how they would like to be viewed and treated. Increasingly consumers have told their stories or had their stories told through articles and books and other means. Those willing to go beyond clinical description of mental illness and to understand mental illness as it affects real people can find many opportunities to do so. Journals like *Schizophrenia Bulletin* and *Psychiatric Services*, for instance, routinely publish first-person reports by consumers, and increasing numbers of autobiographical books are being written by consumers to describe for others their experiences. I include some of these books in the Resource List. In addition, many organizations listed below—such as the National Mental Health Consumers Self-Help Clearinghouse, the National Empowerment Center, and NAMI—maintain speaker lists of consumers willing (in

fact, eager) to talk to community groups and schools and businesses about mental illness.

5. Monitor media and respond to stigmatizing material. Mass media have substantial power to influence public thinking—that is, either to perpetuate or to reduce misconceptions about mental illness. Changing the typically negative ways those with mental illnesses are portrayed in the films and television shows that reach millions of people on a daily basis is necessary if stigma is to be reduced. When we encounter material in mass media that misrepresents and stigmatizes those with mental illnesses, therefore, we should try to let media professionals know our concerns about those presentations. It is a relatively simple matter to send a letter or e-mail to an editor, TV sponsor, or movie producer, and even if a single letter does not get much of a response (although sometimes one *is* enough), the cumulative effect of many letters has been shown to make an impact. In addition, a number of organizations, included on the Resource List below, both contact media about stigmatizing (as well as occasional positive) portrayals and provide assistance to "stigmabusters" in determining whom to write to and what to say.

6. Speak up about stigma. When someone we know misuses a psychiatric term (such as schizophrenia), we can tactfully let them know about the inaccuracy and educate them about the correct meaning. When someone disparages a person with mental illness, tells a joke that ridicules mental illness, or makes disrespectful comments about mental illness, we can let them know that this is hurtful and that, as consumers or mental health advocates, we find such comments offensive and harmful. Although sometimes speaking up in this way may be awkward or intimidating, it is also empowering, as consumers who have done so have discovered.

7. Watch our language. Most of us, including mental health professionals, mental health advocates, and mental health consumers use terms and expressions related to mental illness that may perpetuate stigma. We use psychiatric terms to disparage; for example, we complain about aggressive drivers by calling them "lunatics." We also depersonalize sufferers of mental illness by referring to them generically as "the mentally ill" or by referring to individuals as their disease ("a schizophrenic"). We can avoid contributing to stigma by

avoiding such language and by using what is known as "People First language" to refer to persons, individuals, or people with mental illnesses. The Resource List below includes brochures and handouts that discuss the use of People First language and provide other suggestions for less stigmatizing language that we and others may be encouraged to use.

8. Talk openly about mental illness. The more mental illness remains hidden, the more people believe it is shameful and needs to be concealed. Talking about one's own mental illness or the illness of a loved one can help to counteract the negative attitudes the public possesses. Letting others see real people with mental illnesses—people other than those who make the news with dramatic acts or who appear disheveled on the streets, people who are resourceful, articulate, and creative, people who are familiar already as valued friends or coworkers, people who do *not* fit the public stereotype—is a powerful way to fight stigma. In addition, as consumers observed, talking openly about their mental illnesses can be empowering for individuals with those illnesses and help to remove the internalized stigma they feel. Some organizations on the Resource List below provide support and opportunities for consumers and their families to speak out about their illnesses.

9. Provide support for organizations that fight stigma. The Resource List includes many organizations devoted to education, research, and advocacy concerning mental illness. The influence and effectiveness of the organizations advocating for better treatment and greater acceptance of mental illness depend, to some extent, on membership size and adequacy of finances. They also rely heavily on the effort and passion of their volunteer members. We can contribute to the fight against stigma, then, by joining, volunteering our time and effort, or, if nothing else, donating money to these organizations so that they can continue their work.

10. Demand change from your elected representatives. Policies that perpetuate stigma—from poorer health insurance coverage of mental illness than physical illness to limited funding for research into the causes and treatments of mental illness to inadequate budgets for public mental health services—can be changed if enough people let their representatives know that they want such change. Many

organizations included on the Resource List are actively involved in efforts to generate legislative change; they provide citizens with information on key mental health issues and policies as well as the names of legislators to contact.

Resource List

Books for learning more about mental illnesses
Helping Someone with Mental Illness. Carter, Rosalynn, and Susan
    K. Golant. Random House, 1998.
    This book by the former first lady provides straightforward, lay-oriented information on the major mental illnesses and their treatment. It also offers advice on coping for caregivers and suggestions for helping to erase stigma.

Manic-Depressive Illness. Goodwin, Frederick, and Kay Jamison, eds.
    Oxford University Press, 1990.
This comprehensive book presents information about bipolar or manic-depressive disorder, summarizes the extensive research literature, discusses advances in treatment, and includes the perspectives of those who have had the disorder.

Surviving Mental Illness. Hatfield, Agnes B., and Harriet P. Lefley.
    Guilford Press, 1993.
Two of the early leaders of the family advocacy movement describe the manifestations of schizophrenia and consider the disorder from the perspectives of the individual with the disorder, the family, and the community. The book also highlights aspects of adaptation and recovery.

The Boy Who Couldn't Stop Washing. Rapoport, Judith. E.P. Dutton,
    1989.
This brief book, focusing on obsessive-compulsive disorder, offers both individual stories and general information on OCD causes and treatment.

Surviving Schizophrenia. Torrey, E. Fuller. HarperPerennial, 1995.

This manual for caregivers, now in its third edition, focuses on schizophrenia; the book explains both how its symptoms appear to others and how they are experienced by the individual with the disorder. It also discusses treatment and caregiving issues and contains suggestions for how to advocate and to reduce stigma.

Books for Learning More about the Personal Experiences of People with Mental Illnesses

On the Edge of Darkness. Cronkite, Kathy. Bantam Doubleday, 1994.

The daughter of Walter Cronkite, also a journalist, discusses her experience of depression. She also interviews other accomplished people about their depressions. Contributors include Jules Feiffer, Kitty Dukakis, Rona Barrett, Rod Steiger, and Joan Rivers.

An Unquiet Mind. Jamison, Kay Redfield. Alfred A. Knopf, 1995.

Kay Jamison, a respected therapist and researcher on manic-depressive disorder, discusses her own bipolar illness. She describes the course of her disorder, her personal reactions to it—including fears about how it would affect her credibility as a mental health professional—and her treatment.

Daughter of the Queen of Sheba: A Memoir. Lyden, Jacki. Houghton Mifflin, 1997.

Ms. Lyden, an award-winning National Public Radio correspondent, describes her growing up with a mother with bipolar disorder. The book conveys not only the difficulties of having a mother with this kind of illness, but also how such an illness need not diminish love between parent and child.

Undercurrents: A Life Beneath the Surface. Manning, Martha. Harper Collins, 1994.

In this short book, filled with poignant anecdotes and sharp wit, a clinical psychologist describes her own experience of depression and the stereotypes even she, a mental health professional, had to overcome.

A Beautiful Mind. Nasar, Sylvia. Simon & Schuster, 1998.

This book tells the story of John Nash, a mathematics prodigy who was awarded a 1994 Nobel Prize in Economics for his influential early efforts, but whose work was interrupted for more than twenty years by schizophrenia. The story of his life, his accomplishments, and his struggle with and recovery from schizophrenia are told in moving detail.

Imagining Robert: My Brother, Madness, and Survival. Neugeboren, Jay. William Morrow, 1997.

The author talks about his close relationship with a brother who developed schizophrenia. The book reveals his inspiring and continuing commitment to his brother, Robert, despite the obstacles posed by both his brother's severe illness and the inadequate treatment system they encountered.

The Quiet Room. Schiller, Lori, and Amanda Bennett. Warner Books, 1994.

Lori Schiller describes her courageous struggle with schizophrenia, including its onset during her high school and college years and her successful recovery with the help of new medications. The book also contains chapters by Ms. Schiller's parents and brother, in which they talk about their reactions to the disorder.

Darkness Visible. Styron, William. Random House, 1990.

In this small but powerful book, the Pulitzer Prize–winning author describes his plunge into depression and helps readers to understand how depression can make even the most successful life bleak and joyless.

Books for Learning More about the Problem of Stigma

Stigma and Mental Illness. Fink, Paul Jay, and Alan Tasman, eds. American Psychiatric Press, 1992.

This book contains a series of papers that came out of a 1989 American Psychiatric Association annual meeting, the theme of which was "Overcoming Stigma." The papers discuss societal, historical, and institutional issues of stigma and include narratives from consumers themselves.

Media Madness: Public Images of Mental Illness. Wahl, Otto. Rutgers
    University Press, 1995.
Media Madness explores the mass media depiction of mental illness
and the stigmatizing effects of common stereotypes. It includes many
examples of films, television shows, and novels that depict mental
illness, usually in unfavorable ways, and describes efforts underway
to improve media portrayal of mental illness.

Organizations that Fight Stigma

The Carter Center Mental Health Program, headed by former
first lady and longtime mental health advocate Rosalynn Carter,
works toward reducing stigma and improving mental health care.
The Mental Health Program, for example, sponsors an annual symposium that brings together representatives from most major mental
health groups in the United States to discuss topics of current interest. The Rosalynn Carter Mental Health Journalism Fellowships were
begun in September 1997. This program selects five journalists each
year for funding and mentoring; they generate projects that will provide the public with accurate information about mental illness in
published articles, video news reports, or other media sources. In
addition, the Carter Center presents and distributes videotapes of
panel discussions on various topics as part of its Conversations at
the Carter Center series; one such conversation on mental illness
stigma featured actor Rod Steiger, a sufferer of depression, and au-
thor/journalist Kathy Cronkite. One can learn more about the Carter
Center's mental health activities by contacting the Carter Center
Mental Health Program, One Copenhill, 453 Freedom Parkway, Atlanta, GA, 30307, 404–420–5109 or by visiting their web site (http://
www.cartercenter.org/mentalhealth.htm).

The Center for Mental Health Services (CMHS) of the U.S.
Department of Health and Human Services is mandated to help improve treatment and support services for persons with serious mental illnesses. It operates the Knowledge Exchange Network (KEN),
through which internet users can access extensive information about
mental illnesses, treatment programs, and mental health policies
(http://www.mentalhealth.org). A CMHS brochure, *Before You Label People, Look at Their Contents*, addresses the issue of negative

stereotyping of people with mental illnesses. Contact the National Mental Health Services Knowledge Exchange Network at P.O. Box 42490, Washington, DC, 20015 (1–800–789–2647).

The Erasing the Stigma (ETS) program, begun in 1991 in Mission Valley, California, attacks stigma through work with Rotary Clubs across the country. The ETS program makes presentations to educate Rotarian business leaders about both mental illness itself and about the potential of people with such mental illnesses to be productive employees; ETS then follows up those presentations with efforts to get business leaders to increase their hiring of qualified mental health consumers. Those interested in learning more can write to ETS at 2047 El Cajon Blvd., San Diego, CA, 92104, or call 1–619–543–0412.

NAMI (formerly known as the National Alliance for the Mentally Ill) is one of the largest mental health advocacy groups in the country, with more than 200,000 members and 1,200 state and local affiliates. Most of its members are relatives of people with severe mental illnesses, but the numbers of consumers within the organization is increasing. NAMI provides and helps establish support groups for family members, produces and distributes information about mental illnesses and their treatments, advocates at the local, state, and national levels for policies and resources to improve care for mental illness, and attacks stigma and discrimination. Among their educational materials are a science and treatment kit that contains information, designed for public presentation, concerning what is known about the causes and treatments of serious mental illnesses, and a consumer-produced teaching package about schizophrenia, called "Living with Schizophrenia," that includes an eighteen-minute video, slides, and a discussion guide. In 1995, NAMI began a multiyear Campaign to End Discrimination that includes both high-level lobbying (e.g., for health insurance parity) and grassroots efforts to monitor and respond to stigmatizing depictions of mental illness. Those seeking information can write to NAMI (200 N. Glebe Road, Suite #1015, Arlington, VA, 22203), call their toll-free Helpline (1–800–950–6264), or visit their internet website (http://www.nami.org:80/index.html).

The National Institute of Mental Health (NIMH) is a federal

agency that provides support for research that seeks to understand, treat, and prevent mental illnesses. NIMH also communicates information about psychiatric disorders to scientists, clinicians, news media, and the public. Its Depression: Awareness, Recognition, and Treatment (D/ART) program, a multiyear effort to educate both the public and professionals about depression and its effective treatment, has been followed with a similar program focused on anxiety disorders. Information about these programs and other NIMH efforts can be obtained by contacting the Public Inquiries Office at 6001 Executive Blvd., Room 8184, MSC 9663, Bethesda, MD, 20892–9663 (301–443–4513) or through their website (http://www.nimh.nih.gov). For information on anxiety and depression, call NIMH Information Line (1–800–421–4211).

The National Mental Health Association (NMHA) heads a network of more than 340 state and local affiliates dedicated to improving public knowledge of mental illness and advocating for improved mental health resources. Among its activities are publication and distribution of information brochures about mental health topics (including one on "Stigma: Awareness and Understanding of Mental Illness"), sponsorship of nationwide depression screening days, and coordination of Mental Health Month public education efforts in May of each year. In addition, the National Mental Health Association has begun a Stigma Watch program through which it monitors and responds to media depictions of mental illness, with the help of its many volunteer members and affiliates. The NMHA is located at 1021 Prince Street, Alexandria, VA, 22314, 703–684–7722, has a toll-free number for its Stigma Watch Line (1–800–969–6642), and maintains an internet website (http://www.nmha.org/index.html).

The National Stigma Clearinghouse is a small but effective organization that focuses on monitoring and responding to stigmatizing portrayals of mental illness in the mass media. The Clearinghouse, begun in 1990, receives material from "stigmabusters" across the country and contacts offending media professionals to let them know of the concerns about their presentations. The Clearinghouse also provides suggestions (as well as addresses and phone numbers) for others to respond to media portrayals and occasionally issues "Stigma Alerts" urging widespread response to particular depictions.

Furthermore, the Clearinghouse has developed and/or acquired information materials which can be sent to people in the media for further education about the issues of concern (e.g., an Information for Writers guide). The National Stigma Clearinghouse can be reached at 245 Eighth Avenue, Suite 213, New York, NY, 10011 (212–255–4411).

Organizations Run By and For Consumers

The National Depressive and Manic-Depressive Association (NDMDA) is an organization run by and for people with depressive and manic-depressive disorders. Begun in 1986, it now has a network of 275 chapters and support groups across the United States. Its stated goals are to educate about depressive disorders, foster self-help for consumers, advocate for needed research, and eliminate stigma and discrimination.[1] Information about NDMDA can be obtained from the association's headquarters at 730 Franklin Street, Suite 501, Chicago, IL, 60610–3562 (1–800–826–3632). Their web address is: http://www.ndmda.org.

The National Empowerment Center's stated mission is "to carry a message of recovery, empowerment, hope, and healing to people who have been diagnosed with mental illness."[2] The center provides a national directory of mutual support groups, education to providers from a consumer perspective, and information on a variety of mental health topics. It also arranges for consumers to speak to interested groups to help them better understand mental illness. Its address is 20 Ballard Road, Lawrence, MA, 01843 (1–800–769–3728). On the internet, information about the Center can be found at http://www.concentric.net/~Power2u.

The National Mental Health Consumers Self-Help Clearinghouse provides information and referral services for mental health consumers, consultation for self-help projects, training conferences, and publications for consumers on how to help themselves, including advice on fighting stigma. The Clearinghouse is headquartered at 1211 Chestnut Street, Suite 1000, Philadelphia, PA, 19107 (1–800–553–4539) and maintains its own internet site at http://www.mhselfhelp.org.

The Obsessive-Compulsive Foundation is an international organization of people with obsessive-compulsive disorder (OCD) and their families, friends, and treatment providers. Founded in 1986, its goals are to educate the public about OCD, support those afflicted with this disorder, and encourage research related to OCD.[3] Like other consumer organizations, it also attempts to combat stigma by providing information to reduce public misconceptions. The OCD Foundation can be reached at P.O. Box 70, Milford, CT, 06460–0070 (203–878–5669) or through its website at http://www.ocfoundation. org.

Miscellaneous Additional Resources

Stigma: Language Matters is a colorful, one-page information sheet that identifies the kinds of terms that stigmatize those with mental illnesses and offers alternatives, including an emphasis on People First language to refer to those with psychiatric disorders. This information sheet was developed and can be obtained from The Anti-Stigma Project, 1512 South Edgewood Street, Suite C, Baltimore, MD, 21227.

What Do We Know about Mental Illness and Violence? is a brochure that addresses one of the most damaging stereotypes of mental illness, the idea that it is associated with violence. The brochure contains a consensus statement prepared by some leading experts on the relationship between mental illness and violence; it is a helpful handout or enclosure in trying to help others understand the inaccuracy of fears of people with mental illnesses. Copies may be obtained from Policy Research Associates, 262 Delaware Avenue, Delmar, NY, 12054.

The Stigma of Mental Illness: A Curriculum Video and Training Guide is a teaching tool developed by Boston psychiatrist Kenneth Duckworth. The fifteen- to twenty-minute video includes clips from movies and television shows demonstrating negative stereotypes of mental illness and then addresses those stereotypes. In addition to the video, there are discussion suggestions and a set of questions to be asked before and after the video to assess learning. Although developed for use in the education of medical students, it would be appropriate for school and community audiences of any kind. The video may be obtained through Dr. Duckworth at Massachusetts Mental Health Center, 74 Fenwood Road, Boston, MA, 02115 (617–734–1300).

The *Voices of an Illness* series are radio programs in which both consumers who have mental illnesses and mental health experts on those illnesses discuss specific illnesses. There are three programs, all of which have played on National Public Radio: one on depression, narrated by Rod Steiger (himself a sufferer from depression), one on manic-depressive disorder, narrated by Patty Duke (who has had manic-depressive disorder), and one on schizophrenia, narrated by Jason Robards (whose wife experienced schizophrenia). These tapes may be obtained through Lichtenstein Creative Media, Inc., 105 West 77th Street #5C, New York, NY, 10024 (212–496–8800).

Finally, I have been developing my own internet website, *Otto Wahl's Home Page and Resource Guide for Stigma Busters*, which includes information, articles, "stigma alerts," and links to other internet sites that may be of interest to those wishing to participate in efforts to reduce stigma. This site may be visited at http://mason.gmu.edu/~owahl/INDEX.HTM.

Stigma, as feedback from consumers has suggested, is a pervasive and continuing problem; however, it is not a problem that we must accept as inevitable and unchangeable. Our actions and our involvement in change efforts can—and, I believe, are already starting to—make a difference. I hope that those who read this book will make good use of the resources presented in this chapter to help bring an end to the destructive stigma and discrimination too often faced by people with mental illnesses.

Appendix A

Characteristics of

Survey Participants

(N = 1,388)*

Geographical source

States represented:	50
Number of different zip codes:	773
Most respondents:	
State: California	(95)
City: Milledgeville, GA	(60)

Distribution source

NAMI *Advocate*:	881	(64%)
Consumer Council:	268	(19%)
Internet:	161	(12%)
Other:	74	(5%)

Gender

Females:	781	(56%)
Males:	546	(40%)
Unknown:	61	(4%)

Age

Range = 12–94
Mean = 41.94

Marital status

Single, never married:	591	(43%)
Married:	364	(26%)
Divorced:	318	(23%)
Widowed:	34	(2%)
Unknown:	81	(6%)

Race

Caucasian:	1088	(78%)
African-American:	131	(9%)
Hispanic:	21	(2%)
Asian:	7	(0.5%)
Other:	41	(3%)
Unknown:	100	(7%)

Educational level

Did not complete high school:	165	(12%)
Completed high school:	237	(17%)
Attended, but did not complete, college:	376	(27%)
Completed college:	309	(22%)
Graduate/professional degree:	237	(17%)
Unknown:	64	(5%)

Employment status

Never employed:	40	(3%)
Not employed, but worked previously:	640	(46%)
Employed part-time:	276	(20%)
Employed full-time:	273	(20%)
Unknown:	159	(12%)

Diagnosis   Age at first diagnosis

Bipolar disorder:	350	(25%)	Range = 0–75
Schizophrenia:	248	(18%)	Mean = 25.9
Major depression:	212	(15%)	Mode = 18
Schizoaffective disorder:	74	(5%)	
Multiple diagnoses:	192	(14%)	
Other:	73	(5%)	
Unknown:	239	(17%)	

Number of hospitalizations

Never been hospitalized:	231	(17%)
Hospitalized 1 to 5 times:	609	(43%)
Hospitalized 6 to 20 times:	330	(24%)
Hospitalized 21 to 30 times:	32	(2%)
Hospitalized more than 30 times:	20	(1%)
Unknown:	166	(12%)

Range = 0–98
Mean = 5.7

Current living situation

Independent living in home or apartment:	852	(61%)
Living with parents/other family members:	222	(16%)
Semi-independent living in supervised home/apartment:	158	(11%)
Currently under hospital care:	12	(1%)
No current residence:	4	(0.3%)
Other:	34	(1%)
Unknown:	106	(8%)
Indicated a willingness to be interviewed	847	(61%)
Provided additional written material (elaborations)	451	(33%)

*NOTE: Not all respondents answered all questions. Percentages, nevertheless, are based on the total number of respondents (1,388) in the survey.

Appendix B

Survey Questionnaire

Dear mental health consumer:

We are interested in learning more about how people with identified mental illnesses are treated by others in the community. Rather than do this by asking members of the general public what *they* think about people with psychiatric disorders, as most research studies have done, we would like to hear directly from consumers of mental health services about their personal experiences. Thus, we are asking that you fill out the attached questionnaire concerning your experiences.

The questionnaire will require approximately twenty-five to thirty minutes of your time to complete and is anonymous in the sense that you do not have to include your name. At the end of the questionnaire, however, you will be asked whether you are willing to be interviewed in more detail about your experiences, in which case you would need to provide your name, address, and telephone number. In addition, one section of the questionnaire asks for some personal information. Such information will help us to better understand and interpret results; however, you may omit any items with which you are uncomfortable and still participate in the study.

It is possible that thinking about some of your experiences may prove distressing to you, but there are no other foreseeable risks to you in this study. Your participation, moreover, is voluntary, and you may withdraw from the study at any time and for any reason. Even if you indicate a willingness to be interviewed, you are free to change your mind. There is no penalty for not participating or for withdrawing from the study.

Completed surveys may be mailed directly to us at the address given below. Once information reaches the researchers, it will be treated as confidential. Only the researchers will have access to individual responses, and, although a summary of results will be provided to organizations and individuals requesting it, summaries will *not* identify individuals who have participated without their express written consent.

This study is being conducted by Otto Wahl, Associate Professor of Psychology at George Mason University, and by the National Alliance for the Mentally Ill. Dr. Wahl may be reached at the Department of Psychology, George Mason University, for questions, concerns, or requests for survey results. You may also contact the George Mason University Office of Sponsored Programs if you have any questions regarding your rights as a participant in this research.

This project has been reviewed according to George Mason University procedures governing your participation in this research.

Otto Wahl
Department of Psychology
George Mason University
Fairfax, VA 22030

*A Note about Terms: We recognize that people identified as having psychiatric disorders use many different terms to describe themselves—consumer of mental health services, psychiatric survivor, patient, person with neurobiological brain disorder, and recipient of mental health treatment, among others—and that no one term is agreed upon by all. This survey, for the sake of simplicity, will use primarily the single term "consumer."

Section A: Stigma

Please indicate (by circling the appropriate choice) the extent to which you have experienced any of the following. Remember to base your answers on *your own personal experiences*:

1. I have avoided telling others outside my immediate family that I am a consumer.*

Never   Seldom   Sometimes   Often   Very Often

2. I have been treated as less competent by others when they learned I am a consumer.

Never   Seldom   Sometimes   Often   Very Often

3. Friends who learned I am a consumer have been understanding and supportive.

Never   Seldom   Sometimes   Often   Very Often

4. I have been shunned or avoided by others when it was revealed that I am a consumer.

Never   Seldom   Sometimes   Often   Very Often

5. I have been in situations where I have heard others say unfavorable or offensive things about consumers and their illnesses.

Never   Seldom   Sometimes   Often   Very Often

6. I have been advised to lower my expectations for accomplishments in life because I am a consumer.

Never   Seldom   Sometimes   Often   Very Often

7. I have been treated fairly by others who know I am a consumer.

Never   Seldom   Sometimes   Often   Very Often

8. I have seen or read things in the mass media (e.g., television, movies, books) about consumers and their illnesses which I find hurtful or offensive.

Never   Seldom   Sometimes   Often   Very Often

9. I have worried that others will view me unfavorably because I am a consumer.

Never   Seldom   Sometimes   Often   Very Often

Section B: Discrimination

In this section, we are interested in whether you have been discriminated against as a result of your psychiatric disorder. Please keep in mind that discrimination involves denial of opportunities *on grounds unrelated to your competencies* or level of functioning. If you are turned down for a job, for example, because your illness or symptoms *are* interfering with your ability to fulfill the job requirements, that may not be discrimination. On the other hand, if you are turned down simply on the basis of your having had a mental illness or mental health treatment, without regard to your current abilities, that *would* be considered discrimination. Please keep this distinction in mind as you respond to the following items by circling the response which best fits *your* experience.

1. I have been turned down for a job for which I was qualified when it was revealed that I am a consumer.

Never   Seldom   Sometimes   Often   Very Often

2. I have been denied mental health treatment because my health insurance was insufficient for me to pay the cost of treatment.

Never   Seldom   Sometimes   Often   Very Often

3. I have had difficulty renting an apartment or finding other housing when my status as a consumer was known.
Never   Seldom   Sometimes   Often   Very Often

4. I have been denied educational opportunities (for example, acceptance into schools or education programs) when it was revealed that I am a consumer.
Never   Seldom   Sometimes   Often   Very Often

5. I have been excluded from volunteer or social activities outside the mental health field when it was known that I am a consumer.
Never   Seldom   Sometimes   Often   Very Often

6. I have been excluded from volunteer or other activities within the mental health field when it was known that I was a consumer.
Never   Seldom   Sometimes   Often   Very Often

7. Co-workers or supervisors at work were supportive and accommodating when they learned I am a consumer.
Never   Seldom   Sometimes   Often   Very Often

8. I have been turned down for health insurance coverage on the basis of my mental health treatment history.
Never   Seldom   Sometimes   Often   Very Often

9. I have been denied a passport, driver's license, or other kind of permit when I revealed I am a consumer.
Never   Seldom   Sometimes   Often   Very Often

10. I have had the fact that I am a consumer used against me in legal proceedings (such as child custody or divorce disputes).
Never   Seldom   Sometimes   Often   Very Often

11. I have been treated with kindness and sympathy by law enforcement officers when they learned that I am a consumer.
Never   Seldom   Sometimes   Often   Very Often

12. I have avoided indicating on written applications (for jobs, licenses, housing, school, etc.) that I am a consumer for fear that information will be used against me.
Never   Seldom   Sometimes   Often   Very Often

Section C: Elaboration

Please use this space, if you wish, to explain or elaborate upon any of the responses to the previous questions.

Are there any other ways you have been treated differently (good *or* bad) once others learned you have had mental health treatment? Please explain.

Section D: Background Information

Please provide the following information about yourself by filling in the blank or circling the appropriate answer.

Date of birth: _____ Age: _____

Sex: Male   Female

Marital status: Married   Divorced   Widowed   Single/Never Married

Race: Caucasian/white African-American Hispanic Asian Other

Highest level of education:
    Graduate or professional degree
    Completed college
    Attended but did not complete college
    Completed high school
    Did not complete high school, but completed school through grade _____

What is your current employment status?
    Employed full-time as _____
        since _____
    Employed part-time as _____
        since _____
    Not currently employed, but worked previously as _____
        from _____ to _____
    Never been employed

Nature of mental illness/diagnosis (if known): _____

At what age were you first diagnosed as having a mental illness?_____

Have you ever been treated in a psychiatric hospital?   Yes   No
    If yes, how many hospitalizations have you had? _____

Have you ever been treated through a psychiatric outpatient service?
   If yes, how long were you in treatment? _____

What is your current living situation?
   Independent living in home or apartment
   Semi-independent living in supervised home or apartment
   Living with parents or other family members
   Currently under hospital care
   No current residence
   Other (please explain) _____

We would like to talk further with some of the people filling out this survey in order to get a fuller picture of what they have experienced. IF YOU WOULD BE WILLING TO BE INTERVIEWED CONCERNING YOUR EXPERIENCES, PLEASE READ, SIGN, AND RETURN THE FOLLOWING PAGE WITH YOUR QUESTIONNAIRE. A member of our research team may contact you within the next few months for the interview (although not everyone will be interviewed). If you do *not* wish to be interviewed, simply leave the form blank.

Consent to Be Interviewed

As indicated on the questionnaire you completed, we would like to talk to you further about your experiences. Talking to people, we think, will help us to get a fuller and richer understanding of what consumers have experienced in their lives.

The interview would be conducted by telephone or, when convenient, in person, and would take between 30 and 60 minutes. Interviewers will ask you to elaborate on the experiences you reported on the questionnaire. In particular, interviewers will ask you about specific instances—what happened, how you reacted, how you coped with those experiences—and about some of your general opinions concerning mental illness stigma.

Interviews (including telephone ones) will be tape recorded and later transcribed by graduate students who are part of the research team. Only members of the research team will have access to interview tapes and transcriptions. In addition, interview tapes and transcriptions will be identified and stored by code numbers, and the connection of code numbers with personal identification will be filed separately from tapes and transcriptions. Interview tapes and transcriptions will be retained in locked files until they have been fully analyzed and summarized, after which time they will be destroyed or erased.

Interview material (and material from the previous questionnaire) will be used as the basis of scientific reports—in articles, books, and/or oral presentations, but generally in terms of group summaries rather than individual responses. Specific interview statements may be reported verbatim in research reports, but no names will be attached to these statements without your written permission to do so.

As with the questionnaire, it is possible that thinking about and discussing your experiences may be distressing to you, but there are no other foreseeable risks to you in this interview. Your participation is voluntary. You are free to decline the interview and you may withdraw from or discontinue the interview at any time and for any reason.

If you are willing to be interviewed, we will need you to sign below and to return this form with your questionnaire. Once we have received the signed form, a representative from our research team will call to arrange for the interview.

I HAVE READ AND UNDERSTOOD THE ABOVE INFORMATION CONCERNING MY INTERVIEW PARTICIPATION IN RESEARCH ON MENTAL HEALTH CONSUMERS' EXPERIENCES AND I AM WILLING TO BE INTERVIEWED AS PART OF THAT RESEARCH.

_____   _____   _____

Name (please print)   Signature   Date

_____   _____ _____   _____

Street Address   State   Zip   Phone Number

Appendix C

Characteristics of

of Interviewees

(N = 100)*

Geographical source

States represented:	40
Number of different zip codes:	98
Most respondents: California	(7)

Gender

Females:	71
Males:	29

Marital status

Single, never married:	31
Married:	30
Divorced:	36
Widowed:	2

Distribution source

NAMI *Advocate*:	74
Consumer Council:	17
Internet:	9

Age

Range = 12–94	
Mean = 41.94	

Race

Caucasian:	84
African-American:	9
Hispanic:	0
Asian:	0
Other:	5

Educational level

Did not complete high school:	2
Completed high school:	11
Attended, but did not complete, college:	33
Completed college:	30
Graduate/professional degree:	24

Employment status

Never employed:	1
Not employed, but worked previously:	55
Employed part-time:	22
Employed full-time:	21

Diagnosis		**Age at first diagnosis**
Bipolar disorder:	28	Range = 6–55
Schizophrenia:	17	Mean = 25.5
Major depression:	16	Mode = 20
Schizoaffective disorder:	3	
Multiple diagnoses:	29	
Other:	4	

Number of hospitalizations

Never been hospitalized:	14
Hospitalized 1 to 5 times:	44
Hospitalized 6 to 20 times:	35
Hospitalized 21 to 30 times:	2
Hospitalized more than 30 times:	3

Range = 0–98
Mean = 7.2

Current living situation

Independent living in home or apartment:	77
Living with parents/other family members:	19
Semi-independent living in supervised home/apartment:	2
Currently under hospital care:	0
No current residence:	1
Other:	1

*NOTE: Not all respondents answered all demographic questions on the survey. Thus, totals do not always equal 100.

Appendix D

Responses to Stigma

Items (N = 1,388)*

Statement	Never	Seldom	Sometimes	Often	Very often
I have worried that others will view me unfavorably because I am a consumer.	145 (10%)	129 (9%)	313 (23%)	343 (25%)	432 (31%)
I have been in situations where I have heard others say unfavorable or offensive things about consumers and their illnesses.	132 (10%)	157 (11%)	390 (28%)	367 (26%)	328 (24%)
I have seen or read things in the mass media (e.g., television, movies, books) about consumers and their illnesses which I find hurtful or offensive.	138 (10%)	156 (11%)	413 (30%)	337 (24%)	323 (23%)
I have avoided telling others outside my immediate family that I am a consumer.	186 (13%)	154 (11%)	382 (28%)	290 (21%)	360 (26%)

Statement	Never	Seldom	Sometimes	Often	Very often
I have been treated as less competent by others when they learned I am a consumer.	157 (11%)	216 (16%)	478 (34%)	282 (20%)	221 (16%)
I have been shunned or avoided by others when it was revealed that I am a consumer.	247 (18%)	279 (20%)	472 (34%)	235 (17%)	126 (9%)
I have been advised to lower my expectations in life because I am a consumer.	322 (23%)	255 (18%)	395 (29%)	232 (17%)	156 (11%)
I have been treated fairly by others who know I am a consumer.	53 (4%)	158 (11%)	521 (38%)	438 (32%)	195 (14%)
Friends who learned I am a consumer have been supportive and under-standing.	66 (5%)	151 (11%)	500 (36%)	384 (28%)	260 (19%)

*NOTE: Not all respondents answered all questions. Thus, numbers do not sum to 1,388, and percentages do not total 100.

Appendix E

Responses to

Discrimination

Items (N = 1,388)*

Statement	Never	Seldom	Sometimes	Often	Very often
I have avoided indicating on written applications (for jobs licenses, housing, school, etc.) that I am a consumer for fear that information will be used against me.	250 (18%)	89 (6%)	209 (15%)	244 (18%)	525 (38%)
I have been treated with kindness and sympathy by law enforcement officers when they learned that I am a consumer.	380 (27%)	162 (12%)	308 (22%)	181 (13%)	121 (9%)
Co-workers or supervisors at work were supportive and accommodating when they learned I am a consumer.	206 (15%)	200 (14%)	391 (28%)	282 (20%)	158 (11%)
I have been turned down for a job for which I was qualified when it was revealed that I am a consumer.	656 (47%)	162 (12%)	226 (16%)	136 (10%)	71 (5%)

Statement	Never	Seldom	Sometimes	Often	Very often
I have been denied mental health treatment because my health insurance was insufficient for me to pay the cost of treatment.	712 (51%)	162 (12%)	213 (15%)	115 (8%)	109 (8%)
I have been turned down for health insurance coverage on the basis of my mental health treatment history.	755 (54%)	106 (8%)	161 (12%)	92 (7%)	143 (10%)
I have been excluded from volunteer or social activities outside the mental health field when it was known that I was a consumer.	739 (53%)	199 (14%)	217 (16%)	80 (6%)	49 (4%)
I have been excluded from volunteer or other activities within the mental health field when it was known that I was a consumer.	832 (60%)	175 (13%)	173 (13%)	61 (4%)	36 (3%)
I have had the fact that I am a consumer used against me in legal proceedings (such as child custody or divorce disputes).	889 (64%)	84 (6%)	122 (9%)	72 (5%)	80 (6%)
I have had difficulty renting an apartment or finding other housing when my status as a consumer was known.	850 (61%)	138 (10%)	155 (11%)	63 (5%)	41 (3%)

Statement	Never	Seldom	Sometimes	Often	Very often
I have been denied educational opportunities (for example, acceptance into schools or education programs) when it was revealed that I am a consumer.	922 (66%)	134 (10%)	108 (8%)	53 (4%)	36 (3%)
I have been denied a passport, driver's license, or other kinds of permits when I revealed I am a consumer.	1026 (74%)	94 (7%)	80 (6%)	34 (2%)	25 (2%)

*NOTE: Not all respondents answered all questions. Thus, numbers do not sum to 1,388, and percentages do not total 100.

Notes

<u>*Preface*</u>

1. Michael Cooper, "The Client's Always Right, Even If He's Not," *New York Times*, January 4, 1998. "Judge Rejects Kaczynski's Pleas to Change Lawyers; Trial to Begin Today as Unabomber Suspect Loses Attempt to Exclude Defense Arguments About His Mental Health," *Los Angeles Times*, January 8, 1998.
2. "Martha Stewart Mentally Ill," *National Enquirer*, September 2, 1997. Liz Smith, "Martha Stewart: Crazy? Like A Fox," *New York Post*, September 4, 1997.
3. Kathy Cronkite, *On the Edge of Darkness: Conversations About Conquering Depression* (New York: Doubleday, 1994), 10.
4. Peter Finn, "For sleuth of history, another grave mystery," *Washington Post*, June 3, 1996.
5. Robert Boorstin, Comments made as part of a 1993 public education video prepared by NAMI for its annual meeting in Washington, D.C.
6. Barbara E. Brundage, "What I Wanted to Know But Was Afraid to Ask," *Schizophrenia Bulletin* 9 (1983): 583–585.
7. National Institute of Mental Health, "The Stigma of Mental Illness," DHHS Publication no. (ADM) 90–1470. (Washington, DC: U.S. Department of Health and Human Services, 1990).
8. Lee E. Robins, John E. Helzer, Myrna M. Weissman, Helen Orvaschel, Ernest Gruenberg, Jack D. Burke, Jr., and Darrel Regier, "Lifetime Prevalence of Specific Psychiatric Disorders in Three Sites," *Archives of General Psychiatry* 41 (1984): 949–958. Ronald C. Kessler, Katherine A. McGonagle, Shanyang Ahao, Christopher B. Nelson, Michael Hughes, Suzann Exhelman, Hans-Ulrich Wittchen, and Kenneth S. Kendler, "Lifetime and 12–Month Prevalence of DSM-III-R Psychiatric Disorders in the United States," *Archives of General Psychiatry* 51 (1994): 8–19.
9. Andrew Borinstein, "Public Attitudes Toward Persons With Mental Illness," *Health Affairs* 11 (1992): 186–196.
10. Beldon and Russonello, "Report of Findings From a National Survey on Mental Illness," conducted for the National Alliance for the Mentally Ill, March 1996 (photocopy, 1996).
11. Kim T. Mueser, Shirley M. Glynn, Patrick W. Corrigan, and William Baber, "A Survey of Preferred Terms for Users of Mental Health Services," *Psychiatric Services* 47 (1996): 760–761.

12. Although Mueser et al., in their 1996 study of preference for terms, found that only 8 percent of their sample preferred the term "consumer," their sample did not include those advocates who have been most active in struggling with selecting (and setting the trends for) terminology. In addition, the survey was conducted in 1994 and 1995. I believe there has been an increasing trend since that time toward use of the term "consumer" to designate those with psychiatric disorders. Furthermore, we discussed terminology at length with consumer representatives from NAMI and got feedback on this issue in a pilot study of our survey questionnaire. "Consumer" was the term with which the majority (though certainly not all) of the people we consulted were the most comfortable.

13. NAMI was originally an acronym for the organization known as the National Alliance for the Mentally Ill. Because of concerns about the depersonalizing nature of the term "the mentally ill" in their organization's title (but wishing to retain the acronym by which they had become widely known), that organization decided, in 1998, to be known simply as NAMI.

14. Longtime mental health advocates, Agnes Hatfield and Harriet Lefley, for example, have observed that "there are findings from a very few scientific surveys that actually delve into how mental illness is experienced by adequately large and representative samples of [mental health consumers]." Agnes B. Hatfield and Harriet P. Lefley, *Surviving Mental Illness: Stress, Coping, and Adaptation* (New York: Guilford Press, 1993), vii.

2 *Mental Illness Stigma*

1. Susan Sheehan, *Is There No Place on Earth for Me?* (New York: Houghton Mifflin, 1982).
2. *Webster's New Collegiate Dictionary* (Springfield, MA: G. & C. Meriam Company, 1977).
3. Erving Goffman, *Stigma: Notes on the Management of Spoiled Identity* (Englewood Cliffs, NJ: Prentice-Hall, 1963).
4. Stephen C. Ainlay, Gaylene Becker, and Lerita M. Coleman, *The Dilemma of Difference: A Multidisciplinary View of Stigma* (New York: Plenum Press, 1986), 79.
5. Edward E. Jones, Amerigo Farina, Albert H. Hastorf, Hazel Markus, Dale T. Miller, and Robert A. Scott, *Social Stigma: The Psychology of Marked Relationships* (New York: W. H. Freeman, 1984).
6. Goffman, *Stigma*, 3.
7. Thomas Scheff, *Being Mentally Ill: A Sociological Theory* (Chicago: Aldine Publishing, 1966).
8. Ibid.
9. Gregory Zilboorg and George W. Henry, *A History of Medical Psychology* (New York: W. W. Norton, 1969).
10. Ibid., 583–584.
11. Robert Jay Lifton, *The Nazi Doctors: Medical Killing and the Psychology of Genocide* (New York: Basic Books, 1986).
12. Jum C. Nunnally, *Popular Conceptions of Mental Health* (New York: Holt, Rinehart, and Winston, 1961), 51.
13. Ibid., 270–272.
14. Henry J. Steadman, Edward P. Mulvey, John Monahan, Pamela Clark Robbins, Paul S. Appelbaum, Thomas Grisso, Loren Roth, and Eric Silver, "Violence

by People Discharged from Acute Psychiatric Inpatient Facilities and by Others in the Same Neighborhoods," *Archives of General Psychiatry* 55 (1998): 393–401.

15. Otto F. Wahl, *Media Madness: Public Images of Mental Illness* (New Brunswick, NJ: Rutgers University Press, 1995).

16. The Field Institute, "In Pursuit of Wellness, Vol. 4: A Survey of California Adults Regarding Their Health Practices and Interest in Health Promotion Programs" (Report, California Department of Mental Health, Mental Health Promotion Branch, 1984).

17. Otto F. Wahl, "Public vs. Professional Conceptions of Schizophrenia," *Journal of Community Psychology* 15 (1987): 285–291.

18. Mary E. Fraser, "Educating the Public About Mental Illness: What Will It Take to Get the Job Done," *Innovations and Research* 3 (1994): 29–31.

19. Mark Clements, "What We Say About Mental Illness." *Parade Magazine,* October 31, 1993, 3–6

20. James A. Neff and Baqar A. Husaini, "Lay Images of Mental Illness: Social Knowledge and Tolerance of the Mentally Ill," *Journal of Community Psychology* 13 (1985): 3–12.

21. Fraser, "Educating the Public About Mental Illness."

22. Beldon and Russonello, "Report of Findings from a National Survey on Mental Illness," conducted for the National Alliance for the Mentally Ill, March 1996 (photocopy, 1996).

23. John H. Fryer and Leon Cohen, "Effects of Labeling Patients 'Psychiatric' or 'Medical': Favorability of Traits Ascribed by Hospital Staff," *Psychological Reports* 62 (1988): 779–793.

24. Amerigo Farina and Kenneth Ring, "The Influence of Perceived Mental Illness on Interpersonal Relations," *Journal of Abnormal Psychology* 70 (1965): 47–51.

25. Amerigo Farina, Jack Thaw, John D. Lovern, and Dominick Mangone, "People's Reaction to a Former Mental Patient Moving to Their Neighborhood," *Journal of Community Psychology* 2 (1974): 108–112.

26. David L. Rosenhan, "On Being Sane in Insane Places," *Science* 170 (1973): 250–258.

27. Ibid., 255.

28. Ibid.

29. Ibid., 256.

30. Otto Wahl and Rachel Roth, "Television Images of Mental Illness: Results of a Metropolitan Washington Media Watch," *Journal of Broadcasting* 26 (1982): 599–605.

31. Nancy Signorelli, "The Stigma of Mental Illness on Television," *Journal of Broadcasting and Electronic Media* 33 (1989): 325–331.

32. Steadman et al., "Violence by People Discharged from Acute Psychiatric Inpatient Facilities." It should be noted, however, that, when substance abuse was also involved, discharged patients *were* more violent than their community counterparts. The addition of substance abuse greatly increased the rates of violence among *both* patient and nonpatient populations, but violence increased more for those with accompanying psychiatric disorders. Rates varied with different measures of violence used. When a broad definition of "violence," which included threats, and multiple information sources were used, the rate of violence was estimated to be 17.9 percent for patients with a major mental disorder and *without* substance abuse (about the same as for

nonpatients in the same neighborhood), 31.1 percent for people with a major mental disorder *and* substance abuse, and 43 percent for people with other mental disorders *and* substance abuse.

33. John Monahan, "Mental Disorder and Violent Behavior: Perceptions and Evidence," *American Psychologist* 47 (1992): 511–521. John Monahan and Jean Arnold, "Violence by People With Mental Illness: A Consensus Statement by Advocates and Researchers," *Psychiatric Rehabilitation Journal* 19 (1996): 67–70.

34. Signorelli, "The Stigma of Mental Illness on Television." George Gerbner, "Dreams That Hurt: Mental Illness in the Mass Media," in *Proceedings of the First Annual Rosalynn Carter Symposium on Mental Health Policy* (Atlanta: Carter Center, 1985), 8–13.

35. Donald L. Diefenbach, "The Portrayal of Mental Illness on Prime Time Television," *Journal of Community Psychology* 25 (1997): 289–302.

36. George Gerbner, "Casting and Fate: Women and Minorities in Television Drama, Game Shows, and News," in *Communication, Culture, and Community*, edited by Ed Hollender, Coen van der Linden, and Paul Rutten (Bohn: Stafleu van Loghum, 1995).

37. Russell F. Shain and Julie Phillips, "The Stigma of Mental Illness: Labeling and Stereotyping in the News," in *Risky Business: Communicating Issues of Science, Risk, and Public Policy*, edited by Lee Wilkins and Philip Patterson (Westport, CT: Greenwood Press, 1991), 61–74.

38. David D. Day and Stewart Page, "Portrayal of Mental Illness in Canadian Newspapers," *Canadian Journal of Psychiatry* 31 (1986): 813–816.

39. Charles D. Whatley, "Social Attitudes Toward Discharged Mental Patients," *Social Problems* 6 (1958): 313–320.

40. Richard E. Lamy, "Social Consequences of Mental Illness," *Journal of Consulting Psychology* 30 (1966): 454.

41. John L. Tringo, "The Hierarchy of Preference Toward Disability Groups," *Journal of Special Education* 4 (1970): 295–306.

42. Zachary Gussow and George S. Tracy, "Status, Ideology, and Adaptation to Stigmatized Illness: A Study of Leprosy," *Human Organization* 27 (1968): 316–325.

43. Derek L. Philips, "Public Identification and Acceptance of the Mentally Ill," *American Journal of Public Health* 56 (1966): 755–763.

44. Bruce Purvis, Richard Brandt, Connie Rouse, Vera Wilfred, and Lillian M. Range, "Students' Attitudes Toward Hypothetical Chronically and Acutely Mentally and Physically Ill Individuals," *Psychological Reports* 62 (1988): 627–630.

45. Derek L. Philips, "Rejection: A Possible Consequence of Seeking Help for Mental Disorders," *American Sociological Review* 28 (1963): 963–972.

46. Simon Olshansky, Samuel Grob, and Irene T. Malamud, "Employers' Attitudes and Practices in the Hiring of Ex-Mental Patients," *Mental Hygiene* 42 (1958): 391–401.

47. Amerigo Farina and Robert D. Felner, "Employment Interviewer Reactions to Former Mental Patients," *Journal of Abnormal Psychology* 82 (1973): 268–272.

48. Amerigo Farina, Robert D. Felner, and Louis A. Boudreau, "Reaction of Workers to Male and Female Job Applicants," *Journal of Consulting and Clinical Psychology* 41 (1973): 363–372.

49. Kim C. Oppenheimer and Max D. Miller, "Stereotypic Views of Medical Educators Toward Students with a History of Psychological Counseling," *Journal of Counseling Psychology* 35 (1988): 311–314.

50. Stewart Page, "Effects of the Mental Illness Label in Attempts to Obtain Accommodation," *Canadian Journal of Behavioral Science* 9 (1977): 84–90.

51. Beldon and Russonello, "Report of Findings From a National Survey on Mental Illness," Bruce Link, Elmer L. Struening, Michael Rahav, Jo C. Phelan, and Larry Nuttbrock, "On Stigma and Its Consequences: Evidence from a Longitudinal Study of Men with Dual Diagnoses of Mental Illness and Substance Abuse," *Journal of Health and Social Behavior* 38 (1997): 177–190.

52. Patrick W. Corrigan, Brett Buican, and Stanley McCracken, "Can Severely Mentally Ill Adults Reliably Report Their Needs?" *Journal of Nervous and Mental Disease* 184 (1996): 523–529.

53. Julian Rappaport, "Empowerment Meets Narrative: Listening to Stories and Creating Settings," *American Journal of Community Psychology*, 23 (1995): 796.

54. Ibid., 802.

55. Charles A. Rapp, Wes Shera, and Walter Kisthardt, "Research Strategies for Consumer Empowerment of People with Severe Mental Illness," *Social Work* 38 (1993): 730.

56. Ibid., 729.

3 *Reaching Consumers*

1. Jean Campbell and Ron Schraiber, "The Well-Being Project, Mental Health Consumers Speak For Themselves: A Report of a Survey Conducted for the California Department of Mental Health, Office of Prevention" (Sacramento: The California Network of Mental Health Clients, 1989, photocopy).

2. Freedom From Fear, "Public Perceptions of People With Mental Illness" (Staten Island, N.Y.: Freedom From Fear, 1991, photocopy).

3. Nancy J. Herman, "Return to Sender: Reintegrative Stigma-Management Strategies of Ex-Psychiatric Patients," *Journal of Contemporary Ethnography* 22 (1993): 295–330.

4. We actually received more than 1400 completed surveys. However, some were not used either because they were filled out incorrectly or they were filled out by a nonconsumer (e.g., describing the experiences of a relative).

5. These numbers are approximate because identification of source of the survey was sometimes uncertain. For instance, when survey responses came from a day treatment center, we could not be sure that they were distributed by a member of the Consumer Council or by some other interested party.

6. Not all participants responded to all items. Percentages are based on the total number of respondents (1388), however, not on the number responding to the particular item.

7. NAMI, "Results of the 1995 NAMI [internal membership] Survey" (Arlington, VA: NAMI, 1996, photocopy).

8. Ibid.

9. U.S. Department of Commerce, *Statistical Abstract of the U.S. 1997* (Washington, DC: U.S. Government Printing Office, 1997).

10. Ibid.

11. Ibid.

12. E. Fuller Torrey, Karen Erdman, Sidney M. Wolfe, and Laurie M. Flynn, *Care of the Seriously Mentally Ill, Third Edition* (Washington, DC: Public Citizen Research Group, 1990).

13. E. Fuller Torrey, *Out of the Shadows: Confronting America's Mental Illness Crisis* (New York: John Wiley, 1997).

14. Bruce G. Link, "Understanding Labeling Effects in the Area of Mental Disorders: An Assessment of the Effects of Expectations of Rejection," *American Sociological Review* 52 (1987): 96–112. It should be noted that in Link's more recent work (e.g., Link, Struening, Rahav, Phelan, and Nuttbrock, 1997), he has added a section on actual rejection experiences to his stigma measure. That section includes items such as: "Did some of your friends treat you differently after you had been a patient in a mental hospital?" "Have you ever been refused an apartment or a room because you had been a patient in a mental hospital?" "Have you ever been avoided by people because they knew you were hospitalized in a mental hospital?"

15. Lisa Mansouri and David A. Dowell, "Perceptions of Stigma Among the Long-Term Mentally Ill," *Psychosocial Rehabilitation Journal* 13 (1989): 79–91.

16. Walter R. Gove and Terry Fain, "The Stigma of Mental Hospitalization," *Archives of General Psychiatry* 28 (1973): 494–500.

17. Dan E. Weisburd, ed., "Clients," *The Journal of the California Alliance for the Mentally Ill* 3 (1992).

18. NAMI, *The Experiences of Patients and Families: First Person Accounts* (Arlington, VA: National Alliance for the Mentally Ill, 1989).

19. Kay Redfield Jamison, *An Unquiet Mind: A Memoir of Moods and Madness* (New York: Alfred A. Knopf, 1995).

20. Lori Schiller and Amanda Bennett, *The Quiet Room: A Journey Out of the Torment of Madness* (New York: Warner Books, 1994).

21. Martha Manning, *Undercurrents: A Life Beneath the Surface* (New York: HarperCollins, 1994).

22. William Styron, *Darkness Visible: A Memoir of Madness* (New York: Random House, 1990).

23. Kathy Cronkite, *On the Edge of Darkness* (New York: Doubleday Dell Publishing, 1995).

24. Deborah E. Reidy, "Stigma is Social Death: Mental Health Consumers/Survivors Talk About Stigma in Their Lives" (Holyoke, MA: Education for Community Initiatives, 1993, photocopy). Herman, "Return to Sender."

25. Surveys distributed to the different sources differed slightly in the following ways: (1) Because of space limitations, the survey in the NAMI *Advocate* did not provide space for elaboration, as did the survey distributed in other ways, but urged people to attach a separate sheet with their comments. (2) Consent procedures for interviews involved an additional step for those responding via the internet. Internet responders who indicated a willingness to be interviewed were mailed consent forms for signature and return; those who mailed the survey could sign and return a consent form with the questionnaire. (3) There were also slight differences in instructions for return of surveys to fit the distribution method.

26. The difference here was not statistically significant, however, as determined by use of a standard measure (t-test) of mathematical significance.

4 *Isolation and Rejection*

1. Jean Campbell and Ron Schraiber, "The Well-Being Project, Mental Health Clients Speak For Themselves: A Report of a Survey Conducted for the California Department of Mental Health, Office of Prevention" (Sacramento: The California Network of Mental Health Clients, 1989, photocopy).

2. Bruce G. Link, Elmer L. Struening, Michael Rahav, Jo C. Phelan, and Larry Nuttbrock, "On Stigma and Its Consequences: Evidence From a Longitudi-

nal Study of Men with Dual Diagnoses of Mental Illness and Substance Abuse," *Journal of Health and Social Behavior* 38 (1997): 177–190.

3. Louis Harris and Associates, "Public Attitudes Toward People With Disabilities: Conducted for the National Organization on Disability" (New York: National Organization on Disability, 1991, photocopy).

4. Deborah Reidy, "Stigma is Social Death: Mental Health Consumers/Survivors Talk About Stigma in Their Lives," (Holyoke, MA: Education for Community Initiatives, 1993, photocopy).

5 *Discouragement and Lowered Goals*

1. John Nash is a mathematician who has suffered from schizophrenia for more than twenty years. In 1994, he was awarded the Nobel Prize for Economics based on his early work on game theory. His story is described in *A Beautiful Mind* by Sylvia Nasar (New York: Simon and Schuster, 1998). William Styron, the acclaimed author of *Sophie's Choice*, had to seek hospital treatment for severe depression; he tells about this experience in his book, *Darkness Visible* (New York: Random House, 1990). Academy Award–winning actress Patty Duke has achieved her success despite a life-long struggle with bipolar (manic-depressive) disorder, a struggle she describes in *A Brilliant Madness: Living with Manic-Depressive Illness* (New York: Bantam Books, 1992). Lawton Chiles had been elected to the U.S. Senate and was twice elected governor of Florida, the second time despite revelation of a history of treatment for depression.

2. It must be acknowledged here that some confusion between mental illness and mental retardation comes from within the field of psychiatry. Although most clinicians would strongly agree that differentiation between mental illness and mental retardation is appropriate and necessary, the official United States guide to classification of psychiatric disorders, *DSM-IV*, does include mental retardation in its listing of "mental disorders."

3. Esso Leete, "Stressor, Symptom, or Sequelae? Remission, Recovery, or Cure?" *Journal of the California Alliance for the Mentally Ill* 5 (1994): 17.

4. Kay Jamison has talked about her bipolar disorder in a best-selling book, *An Unquiet Mind* (New York: Alfred A. Knopf, 1995), and Fred Frese's story has been recounted numerous places, including the Ohio *Beacon Journal* (Katerine Spitz and Robin Week, "The Odyssey of Fred Frese," *The Beacon Journal*, March 6, 1994), and the *Detroit Free Press* (Patricia Anstett, "Living With Schizophrenia," *Detroit Free Press*, June 18, 1996).

6 *Discrimination*

1. For a good summary of the Americans with Disabilities Act as it applies to psychiatric disabilities, see the background paper produced by the Office of Technology Assessment: "Psychiatric Disabilities, Employment, and the Americans With Disabilities Act" (Washington, DC: U.S. Government Printing Office, 1994).

2. At first glance, the percentage of people reporting job discrimination may seem reassuringly low, but it is important to note that those consumers who indicated no such discrimination were not necessarily doing so because they had been successful in the job market. On the contrary, many consumers were disabled early in their adult lives, live on Social Security or other disability incomes, had never applied for jobs, and thus never faced discrimination.

Such individuals frequently responded to the job discrimination items on the survey by adding "Not Applicable" and/or explaining that they had never been turned down for a job because they had never applied. In addition, 70 percent of our respondents indicated that they had at least sometimes avoided indicating on written applications that they were consumers; this allowed them to escape discriminatory job treatment by concealing what could be the basis for such discrimination. If we had looked only at those persons who had applied for jobs and who did not conceal their illnesses, the percentage who had been turned down for a job would undoubtedly have been much higher.

3. Dorothy Miller and William H. Dawson, "Effects of Stigma on Re-employment of Ex-Mental Patients," *Mental Hygiene* 49 (1965): 281–287.

4. Don Spiegel and Jenny B. Younger, "Life Outside the Hospital: A View From Patients and Relatives," *Mental Hygiene* 56 (1972): 9–20. Bruce G. Link, Elmer L. Struening, Michael Rahav, Jo C. Phelan, and Larry Nuttbrock, "On Stigma and Its Consequences: Evidence From a Longitudinal Study of Men With Dual Diagnoses of Mental Illness and Substance Abuse" *Journal of Health and Social Behavior* 38 (1997): 177–190.

5. Again, the percentage of respondents who did not receive accommodations is lowered by two main factors: many did not work and thus did not need accommodation; and many who worked did not reveal their illnesses or request accommodations. This kind of limitation was true, in fact, for virtually all the discrimination items. Approximately 20 percent of respondents indicated that one or more of the discrimination items were not applicable to them because they had not been involved in the target activity. Another 8 percent made notations to their responses explaining that they had not experienced discrimination because they had not disclosed their illnesses.

6. Not all respondents were in a position to experience discrimination because they did not volunteer. At the same time, it is noteworthy how many consumers apparently did attempt to volunteer their time and energy. Contrary to the perception of consumers as poorly motivated malingerers, as described in chapter 5, many consumers sought out opportunities to contribute to their communities even without financial compensation.

7. Once again, discrimination percentages are reasonably low in part because many consumers did not have to seek housing (living with parents or spouses or in supervised settings provided through mental health programs) and many did not reveal their consumer status to prospective landlords.

8. Link, et al., "On Stigma and Its Consequences."

9. The modest number of people reporting discrimination again may be misleading. Those treated through public mental health facilities or receiving care as part of disability entitlements were not faced with applying for insurance and thus would not have had the experience of being denied. Others had no difficulty obtaining insurance mainly because, as several consumers wrote, they were wise enough to conceal their psychiatric treatment histories.

10. Legal discrimination is probably the best example of how low numbers are misleading. The item related to this type of discrimination was the one most likely to produce notes that it was not applicable because the person had never been involved with the police or the courts and thus had had no opportunity to be treated either fairly or unfairly.

11. A prime example of this belief that those with mental illnesses (and other transgressors) are somehow treated too kindly is the July 20, 1998, issue of *National Review*, the cover of which proclaimed (beside a picture of *Psycho*'s

Norman Bates) "Psycho Babble: How America Indulges the Mentally Ill, Coddles Wife Beaters—And Persecutes Normal Parents." The belief that criminal law "indulges" those with mental illnesses, however, is contradicted by considerable research. Those with mental illnesses, for example, are more likely to be jailed for minor offenses and to spend more time in jail when arrested than those without psychiatric disorders. For more information, see a good account of problems faced by consumers in the criminal justice system by E. Fuller Torrey, Joan Stieber, Jonathon Ezekiel, Sidney M. Wolfe, Joshua Sharfstein, John H. Noble, Laurie Flynn, "Criminalizing the Seriously Mentally Ill" (Washington, DC: Citizens Health Research Group and the National Alliance for the Mentally Ill, 1992).

12. Although many members of the general public believe that the insanity defense is widely used for defendants to escape criminal responsibility and achieve light sentences for serious crimes, research shows that this is not true. In reality, the insanity defense is rarely used and even more rarely successful. Insanity plea acquittees spend substantial time incarcerated, sometimes even longer than they would have if they had been convicted of the (sometimes minor) crimes of which they were accused. For more information, see: Eric Silver, Carmen Cirincione, and Henry J. Steadman, "Demythologizing Inaccurate Perceptions of the Insanity Defense," *Law and Human Behavior* 18 (1994): 63–70.

7 Indirect Stigma

1. Erving Goffman, *Stigma: Notes on the Management of Spoiled Identity* (Englewood Cliffs, NJ: Prentice-Hall, 1963).

2. Some may wonder, if potentially offensive media depictions of mental illness are as common as previous research suggests—e.g., see Otto Wahl, *Media Madness: Public Images of Mental Illness* (New Brunswick, NJ: Rutgers University Press, 1995)—why 22 percent of consumer respondents reported that they had seldom or never seen or read things in the mass media they found hurtful or offensive. It is possible that some individuals do little television or film viewing. It is also likely that "consumers" are not a uniform group; like nonconsumers, they have differing degrees of sensitivity and tolerance, as well as diversity in their opinions about what is hurtful and offensive.

3. Most of television and film, of course, is overly dramatic, not just portrayals of mental illness. As Robert P. Snow has pointed out in his book, *Creating Media Culture* (Beverly Hills, CA: Sage Publications, 1983), attracting and holding a film or television audience requires characters who are both larger than life and easily identifiable. Portraying mental illness in its extreme fits this bill particularly well.

4. Many examples of the media misuse of the term "schizophrenia" are provided in Wahl's *Media Madness*.

5. Consumer fears that portrayals of killers with mental illness may contribute to continuing fear of consumers are supported by research findings that have demonstrated more fearful attitudes following a TV movie about a man who killed his wife while on a pass from a psychiatric hospital (Otto F. Wahl and John Y. Lefkowits, "Impact of a Television Film on Attitudes Toward Mental Illness," *American Journal of Community Psychology* 17 (1989): 521–527) or subsequent to reading a newspaper story about a murder committed by a psychiatric patient (Joann A. Thornton and Otto F. Wahl, "Impact of a Newspaper

Article on Attitudes Toward Mental Illness," *Journal of Community Psychology* 24 (1996): 17–25).

6. George Gerbner, "Casting and Fate: Women and Minorities in Television Drama, Game Shows, and News," in *Communication, Culture, and Community,* edited by Ed Hollender, Coen Van der Linden, and Paul Rutten (Bohn: Stafleu van Loghum, 1995).

7. Nancy Signorelli, "The Stigma of Mental Illness on Television," *Journal of Broadcasting and Electronic Media* 33 (1989): 325–331.

8. Russell F. Shain and Julie Phillips, "The Stigma of Mental Illness: Labeling and Stereotyping in the News," in *Risky Business: Communicating Issues of Science, Risk, and Public Policy,* edited by Lee Wilkins and Philip Patterson (Westport, CT: Greenwood Press, 1991), 61–74.

9. Certainly, there may have been more positive media depictions of mental illness than have been mentioned or than consumers observed. The survey, after all, asked specifically about negative encounters and contained only a general request for positive experiences (in particular, for elaboration about experiences "good or bad").

8 *Impact of Stigma*

1. To identify specific reactions, each interview was read and rated by three different psychology doctoral students at George Mason University. Using a list of possible reactions suggested by our interviewers based on their conversations with consumers, these raters made judgments about the specific reactions being conveyed. Where a specific reaction was clearly communicated, such that two out of the three raters agreed on its presence, that reaction was recorded.

2. Bruce Link, Jerrold Mirotznik, and Francis T. Cullen, "The Effectiveness of Stigma Coping Orientations: Can Negative Consequences of Mental Illness Labeling Be Avoided?" *Journal of Health and Social Behavior* 32 (1991): 302–320.

3. This new emphasis on personal recovery rather than treatment has been described eloquently by William A. Anthony (e.g., in "The Recovery Vision," *Journal of the California Alliance for the Mentally Ill* 5 (1994): 5.

4. Patricia Deegan, "A Letter to My Friend Who Is Giving Up," *Journal of the California Alliance for the Mentally Ill,* 5 (1994): 18.

9 *Strategies and Coping*

1. As William A. Anthony has explained: "Recovery, as we currently understand it, means growing beyond the catastrophe of mental illness and developing new meaning and purpose in one's life. It means taking charge of one's life even if one cannot take complete charge of one's symptoms." See "The Recovery Vision," *Journal of the California Alliance for the Mentally Ill* 5 (1994): 5.

2. Agnes B. Hatfield, "Recovery From Mental Illness," *Journal of the California Alliance for the Mentally Ill* 5 (1994): 6.

3. Freedom From Fear, "Public Perceptions of People With Mental Illness" (Staten Island, NY: Freedom From Fear, 1991, photocopy).

4. Bruce G. Link, Francis T. Cullen, Elmer Struening, Patrick E. Shrout, and Bruce P. Dohrenwend, "A Modified Labeling Theory Approach To Mental

Disorders: An Empirical Assessment," *American Sociological Review* 54 (1989): 400–423.

5. Bruce G. Link, Jerrold Mirotznik, and Francis T. Cullen, "The Effectiveness of Stigma Coping Orientations: Can Negative Consequences of Mental Illness Labeling Be Avoided?" *Journal of Health and Social Behavior* 32 (1991): 302–320.

6. Nancy J. Herman, "Return to Sender: Reintegrative Stigma-Management Strategies of Ex-Psychiatric Patients," *Journal of Contemporary Ethnography* 22 (1993): 295–330.

7. According to Herman, the strategy of "therapeutic disclosure" was almost always perceived to be helpful by those consumers to whom she spoke.

8. Nancy Herman also identified a comparable strategy, which she called "political activism," as commonly used by the consumers in her 1993 Canadian study ("Return to Sender").

9. Many stigma-reduction strategies suggested by consumers in our study are actually being carried out by various mental health and advocacy groups. For instance, the large-scale public education activities about mental illness recommended by consumers is being attempted. The National Institute of Mental Health (NIMH) has sponsored the multiyear, multimedia D/ART (Depression/Awareness, Recognition, and Treatment) program to educate both the public and medical professionals about depression and its treatment. NIMH is also now carrying out a similar public education campaign about anxiety disorders. NAMI is engaged in a nationwide Campaign To End Discrimination, which includes extensive public education materials about severe mental illnesses such as schizophrenia and bipolar disorder. The National Mental Health Association (NMHA) likewise has been carrying out a public education Campaign on Clinical Depression since 1992 and launched an Anxiety Disorders Education Campaign in November 1998.

10. Consumer recommendations about physician education fit with current efforts to accomplish such education. NAMI has a curriculum committee that looks at the curriculum in professional training programs and encourages more extensive, more informed, and more empathetic coverage of mental illness. NIMH and NMHA have focused on physician education in portions of their depression education campaigns. In addition, Kenneth Duckworth, M.D., medical director of the Massachusetts Mental Health Center, has developed a video and training guide specifically about mental illness stigma to be used in medical and other professional training. His curriculum was distributed in 1997 to directors of psychiatric training programs; he has planned additional distribution to programs training social workers, nurses, primary care physicians, and psychologists.

11. In line with consumer suggestions, advocates are pushing efforts to educate journalists about mental illness and to encourage improved news coverage of the topic. The Rosalynn Carter Mental Health Journalism Fellowships, for instance, provide financial support, education, and mentoring for selected journalists to complete projects related to mental illness. Such projects have included newspaper stories about children's mental health and the deficiencies of psychiatric care in prisons, as well as television news stories about the limitations of health insurance for mental health treatment.

12. Prominent people with mental illnesses have appeared on television and radio talk shows, as consumers have recommended; such appearances include people such as Mike Wallace, Kathy Cronkite, and Rod Steiger, all sufferers

from depression. There has been much less success, however, persuading talk show hosts to risk their ratings on "average" citizens who have psychiatric disorders.

13. There have been some excellent documentaries on television concerning mental illness. HBO, for example, has presented *Into Madness: America Undercover Looks at Schizophrenia* in 1989, and, more recently, *Dead Blue: Surviving Depression,* which featured Mike Wallace, Martha Manning, and William Styron discussing their experiences of depression. The latter was shown numerous times in January 1998; it aired at various times during the year that followed. Other programs, including WNET's (New York) one-hour documentary discussion of mental illness stigma, *Unraveling the Myths* in March 1990; a thirty–minute episode of *The Cutting Edge Medical Report* on the Discovery Channel during Fall 1995 which focused on schizophrenia; and WSKG-TV's (Binghamton, New York) 1996 program, *Speaking for Ourselves,* about the self-help and empowerment movement in mental health, have provided consumer-recommended documentary coverage of mental illness. A concern, of course, is that only a limited audience often sees such documentaries, while entertainment features offering mentally ill killers are viewed by millions on a regular basis.

14. There actually had been a Public Service Announcement (PSA) about mental illness that played during National Football League games during the 1987–1988 season (although not during the Super Bowl). Millions of football fans saw Lionel Aldridge, a former defensive end for the Green Bay Packers in their early Super Bowl championships, revealing that he had developed schizophrenia subsequent to his football career.

15. Others agree that it would be helpful for high-ranking politicians to talk about mental illness, and many political figures have indeed discussed it on the news and elsewhere. Tipper Gore, wife of Vice President Al Gore, has been an outspoken advocate for mental health. Florida Governor Lawton Chiles had openly discussed his own treatment for depression. Senators Pete Domenici and Paul Wellstone have revealed that they have relatives with severe mental illnesses and championed legislation to provide better health insurance coverage for those with psychiatric disorders.

16. Both Martha Manning and Kay Jamison are psychotherapists who wrote books about their personal experiences of mental illness (see list of books in chapter 12); it is not known whether there are plans to make either book into a movie. Films about real people with mental illnesses are far more rare than the ubiquitous "psycho-killer" films, although some have been produced. *Call Me Anna,* the 1990 television film about Patty Duke's struggle with bipolar disorder, for example, has been shown numerous times. *Shine,* the story of musician David Helfgott, who returned to performing as a concert pianist after a schizophrenic breakdown, received seven Academy Award nominations in 1997, including best director and best picture, and its star, Geoffrey Rush, won the Oscar for best actor.

17. The ad being referred to was probably a poster developed by NAMI for Mental Illness Awareness Week in 1991 (October 6–13). The poster presented a long list of famous people who have had mental illness and declared that "People with mental illness enrich our lives." On the list were Abraham Lincoln and Winston Churchill, both of whom are known to have been afflicted with depression. Lincoln once declared that "I am now the most miserable man living. If what I feel were equally distributed to the whole human family, there would be not one cheerful face on earth." Churchill referred to

his depression as "the black dog" for the bleakness it brought and the tenacity with which it took hold.

18. People like Kay Jamison, Mike Wallace, Naomi Judd, and Art Buchwald *have* talked openly about their mental illnesses. Some of these individuals, and many others, in fact, were interviewed by Kathy Cronkite, and they tell of their experiences of depression in her book, *On the Edge of Darkness: Conversations about Conquering Depression* (New York: Bantam Doubleday, 1994).

19. As noted previously, Patty Duke's story of her life with bipolar disorder has been told in both an autobiographical book (*A Brilliant Madness*) and a television movie (*Call Me Anna*). Margot Kidder, best known for her portrayal of Lois Lane in the Superman movies, was revealed to have bipolar disorder after an April 1996 incident in which she was reported missing and later discovered in a disheveled state in someone's backyard. Her story was subsequently told in a variety of prominent news sources, including *People Weekly* magazine, *Maclean's*, and "20/20."

20. Consumers will be pleased to know that there *is* an organization like the American Cancer Society that raises money for research into mental illness—the National Alliance for Research on Schizophrenia and Depression (NARSAD). Recognizing the great need for funds for research into the causes and treatments of mental illness, several mental health advocacy groups (NAMI, the National Mental Health Association, the National Depressive and Manic Depressive Association, and the Schizophrenia Research Foundation) established NARSAD specifically to raise funds for mental illness research. Since its inception in 1987, NARSAD has raised and awarded research grants in amounts that exceed 64 million dollars.

21. Legal actions, such as consumers recommended, have been pursued by mental health advocates. NAMI and the National Mental Health Association have strongly advocated for mandated parity (equal coverage of mental and physical health problems) in health insurance, with substantial success. Congress passed limited parity legislation in 1996, and additional bills to require parity in health insurance have been passed or introduced in more than thirty states; see Mental Health Parity Act of 1996, Public Law 204, 104th Cong., (26 September 1996), Title VII, 110 Stat. 2944 (codified at *U.S. Code*, vol. 29, sec. 1185a, and at *U.S. Code*, vol. 42, sec. 300 gg–5). Also, the inclusion of mental disability in the 1990 Americans with Disability Act, along with issuance of specific enforcement guidelines by the Equal Employment Opportunity Commission in March 1997, has enabled thousands of mental health consumers to gain legal redress for job discrimination.

22. Once again, consumer suggestions fit with activities already underway to reduce stigma. There already exist organizations that make it their jobs to identify and respond to stigmatizing information about mental illness. The primary activity of the National Stigma Clearinghouse, for example, is to contact media professionals about stigmatizing (or particularly positive) depictions of mental illness. The National Mental Health Association's Stigma Watch program and NAMI's StigmaBusters Network operate similarly.

23. Those survey participants who reported filing EEOC complaints were not alone. According to a report in the May/June 1997 *NAMI Advocate*, approximately 12.7 percent of all employment discrimination charges filed with the Equal Employment Opportunity Commission under the Americans with Disabilities Act during its first four years (from 1992 to 1996) involved mental or psychiatric disabilities. That represents more than five thousand claims.

24. Speakers' Bureaus and programs in which consumers go to businesses and classrooms to talk about mental illness and about their own experiences with psychiatric disorder do exist. The Breaking the Silence program, developed by a NAMI affiliate in New York, for example, has been for many years bringing information about mental illness to schools in an attempt to counteract stigma. The Erasing the Stigma program, begun in California in 1991, does a similar thing with businesses as its target.
25. Many organizations and advocacy groups—such as NAMI, the National Empowerment Center, the National Mental Health Consumers Self-Help Clearinghouse—maintain lists of consumers willing to speak to students, business executives, reporters, and anyone else interested in learning more about mental illnesses.
26. Shiela M. LaPolla, "Disclosure," *Journal of the California Alliance for the Mentally Ill* 6 (1995): 54.
27. Research has suggested, in fact, that stories of recovery from mental illness are particularly effective in dispelling stigma. See David L. Penn, Kim Guynan, Tamara Daily, William D. Spaudling, Calvin P. Garbin, and Mary Sullivan, "Dispelling the Stigma of Schizophrenia: What Sort of Information Is Best?" *Schizophrenia Bulletin* 20 (1994): 567–578.

10   *Consumer Messages about Mental Illness*

1. Consumer concerns that others see them only in terms of their illness is consistent with psychiatric disorder being a "master trait," as discussed in chapter 2.
2. Consumer requests to be recognized as people primarily who happen secondarily to have a disorder fit with a broader disability movement toward People First language and thought. Individuals with disabilities of all kinds are demanding to be described as "people with" a certain disability—just as we would speak of people with cancer or heart disease (rather than "the cancerous" or the "heart diseased")—a nomenclature that emphasizes their personhood rather than their disabilities. For further discussion of this issue, see Joan Blaska, "The Power of Language: Speak and Write Using 'People First' Language," in *Perspectives on Disability*, 2d ed., edited by Mark Nagler (Palo Alto, California: Health Markets Research, 1993), 25–32; Susan Spaniol and Mariagnese Cattaneo, "The Power of Language in the Helping Relationship," in *Psychological and Social Aspects of Psychiatric Disability*, edited by Leroy Spaniel, Cheryl Gagne, and Martin Kohler (Boston: Center for Psychiatric Services, 1997), 477–484.

11   *Cautions and Limitations*

1. About 40 percent of our consumer survey respondents were employed full-time or part-time. Studies conducted by the National Institute of Mental Health have suggested that the employment rate for people with disorders similar to those in our survey (i.e., with serious mental illnesses such as schizophrenia and bipolar disorder) may be as low as 15 percent.
2. Studies of public attitudes have shown that generic terms like "the mentally ill" or "mental patients" are sufficient to generate consistent social rejection. To be fair, however, we must note that the public has seldom been asked to distinguish among types of mental illness, with most of the stigma

research employing only generic terms that encourage their subjects to think of those with mental illnesses as a uniform group.

3. Early stigma studies also demonstrated that any kind of treatment for psychiatric problems generated rejection, although psychiatric hospitalization was clearly more stigma producing than treatment by a general practitioner or member of the clergy. Derek L. Phillips, "Rejection: A Possible Consequence of Seeking Help For Mental Disorders," *American Sociological Review* 28 (1963): 963–972.

4. Deborah E. Reidy, "Stigma is Social Death: Mental Health Consumers/Survivors Talk About Stigma in Their Lives" (Holyoke, MA: Education for Community Initiatives, 1993, photocopy).

12   *Resources for Fighting Stigma*

1. Goals are those presented in a 1998 brochure of the National Depressive and Manic-Depressive Association.

2. Goals are those articulated in the mission statement of the National Empowerment Center presented on their internet website.

3. Goals are those listed in the mission statement of the Obsessive-Compulsive Foundation (OCF), which appears on the OCF internet website.

Index

About the Author

Otto Wahl received a B.A. in psychology from Wesleyan University and a Ph.D. in clinical psychology from the University of Pennsylvania. He is currently a professor of psychology at George Mason University in Fairfax, Virginia. He is also on the advisory boards of the National Stigma Clearinghouse, the NAMI Campaign to End Discrimination, and the Rosalynn Carter Mental Health Journalism Fellowships. Dr. Wahl has written extensively on stigma and public misunderstanding of mental illness and has made presentations on this topic at numerous mental health conferences as well as on radio and television programs. His previous book, *Media Madness: Public Images of Mental Illness*, which examined the portrayal of mental illness in the mass media, received the Gustavus Myers Award as "an outstanding book on human rights in North America."

DATE DUE

			Printed in USA